ADVANCE PRAISE

"I'm all about finding new ways to hack my fitness, which is why I love Jay Kim's book, Hack Your Fitness! This book will help many people who are looking to lose weight, add muscle or just focus on improving their health."

— DREW MANNING, NEW YORK TIMES BESTSELLING AUTHOR OF FIT2FAT2FIT: THE UNEXPECTED LESSONS FROM GAINING AND LOSING 75 LBS ON PURPOSE

"Hack Your Fitness is exactly what is sounds like, the quickest route to getting in the best shape of your life. What are you waiting for?!"

— DAVE MCCLURE, FOUNDING PARTNER, 500 STARTUPS

"Hack Your Fitness is perfect for very busy, successful people to spend the minimum amount of time necessary to have the best physique of their life."

— NATHAN CHAN, CEO & PUBLISHER, FOUNDR MAGAZINE

"Jay Kim did the hard work to understand fitness so you don't have to."

— DR. JOHN RATEY, ASSOCIATE CLINICAL PROFESSOR OF PSYCHIATRY, HARVARD MEDICAL SCHOOL

"As an entrepreneur who's constantly busy, it's hard to find time to stay fit. Hack Your Fitness is the perfect roadmap for anyone looking to get fit while saving valuable time."

— BENNY LUO, FOUNDER, NEXTSHARK.COM, THE VOICE OF THE GLOBAL ASIAN YOUTH

"The most valuable commodity in the world is time and Jay Kim explains exactly how to make more progress in less time."

— DAVID CHANG, CO-FOUNDER OF CROSSFIT 852, MANAGING PARTNER OF MINDWORKS VENTURES

"As a married, working father of a 6 month old I've been waiting for a book like this to be written. Jay Kim delivers a balanced look at how to streamline your diet and fitness without compromising time at home or placing undue demands on loved ones."

— DR. JASON KANG, DIRECTOR, BLOOD BANKS AT NORTHSHORE UNIVERSITY HEALTHSYSTEM

"Jay Kim's lifestyle solution is perfect for busy people that cannot spend 6 days in the gym."

— DR. ROGER KING, FOUNDING DIRECTOR, THOMPSON CENTRE FOR BUSINESS CASE STUDIES AND THE TANOTO CENTRE FOR ASIAN FAMILY BUSINESS AND ENTREPRENEURSHIP STUDIES AT THE HKUST

"Hack Your Fitness is the solution we've all been waiting for that is simple and sustainable for life!"

— DARYL NG, EXECUTIVE DIRECTOR, SINO GROUP, TOP 10 LARGEST PROPERTY DEVELOPER IN HONG KONG VOTED 'BEST DEVELOPER OVERALL IN HONG KONG' BY EUROMONEY REAL ESTATE SURVEY 2015

"Well-written and thoroughly researched. A must read for every busy entrepreneur!"

"More so than the physical benefits, exercise supports my mental health and is the key to my overall happiness. Working in the startup world, my hours are all over the place, making it nearly impossible to block off time for the gym. Hack Your Fitness provided me with excellent advice for fitting effective exercise into my busy day, keeping my mental health in tip-top shape."

"The best thing I ever did for myself was join Jay's program. I ended up losing 30lbs over the course of 3 months and am now enjoying the benefits of a healthier lifestyle. Nothing in life comes easy, but if you are ready to commit yourself to Jay's plan, you will achieve results. For my colleagues and friends who keep asking how I did it, go pick up Jay's book!"

HACK YOUR FITNESS

HACK YOUR FITNESS

THE HIGH ACHIEVER'S GUIDE TO GETTING RIPPED IN UNDER

3 HOURS A WEEK

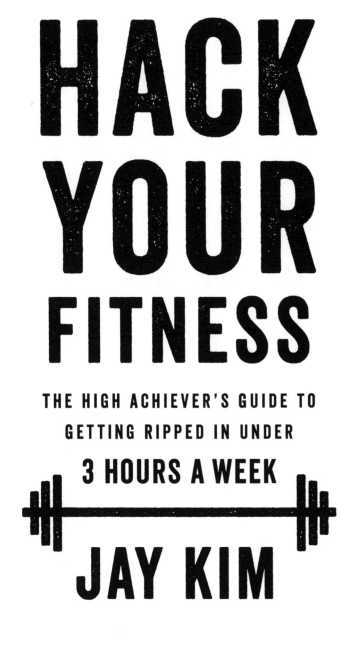

JAY KIM

HACK YOUR FITNESS

The High Achiever's Guide to Getting
Ripped in Under 3 Hours a Week

ISBN   978-1-61961-589-2 *Paperback*
          978-1-61961-590-8 *Ebook*

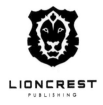

LIONCREST
PUBLISHING

· For Ev ·

CONTENTS

FOREWORD

My lifelong passion for fitness began much earlier than most people.

As a child, I fell in love with racing at the tender age of eight when my father bought me my first go-kart. My dad, who had competed semi-professionally in Canada, offered to retire from racing, sell his car, and invest his time and money into my development as a driver. By the age of fifteen, I was competing in over twenty races a year all across Canada and the United States.

Being a Chinese race car driver in North America was, and still is, not easily marketable. But once I arrived in Asia, I realized how big of an opportunity there was for me in a growing market, especially China. I got my first big break in 2004 when I was offered a spot on a team in the Porsche Carrera Cup Asia.

I went on to race with Porsche for the next six years, winning several championships including three wins at the Macau Grand Prix, which led me to one of the proudest achievements of my career in 2013: a podium finish at 24 Hours of Le Mans, the most historic and prestigious endurance race in the world.

But long before all those championships and podium finishes, my racing career was built on one main foundation—fitness.

As a professional race car driver, I have always considered fitness to be a crucial part of my career. Racing requires a different type of fitness than most other sports. Imagine sitting crouched behind a wheel, driving as fast as you possibly can, for hours straight. Most people are unaware of how physically and mentally demanding racing actually is due to the heat and intense g-forces. Because of this, I trained very hard in a way that I thought was right for me: cardiovascular training, functional movements, full body workouts, but never heavy weight lifting.

I used to train five or six days a week for a few hours at a time. My cardiovascular fitness was superb, but weight gain was always a problem for me. This is something I battled with since I was a child, and because my father was overweight, I simply thought it was bad genetics. I thought I was just dealt a bad hand in life.

To top of it off, my career had me traveling for thirty weeks out of the year. I always tried to "eat clean" when I could and to train as hard as possible. But no matter how hard I tried, my body fat just kept creeping up. In desperation, I even hired personal trainers and dieticians in a bid to try and lean out, but that failed, too.

As a professional athlete and public figure, my image is a big part of my brand. I was constantly on camera for press photos and interviews, but I never really felt confident in my appearance.

I met Jay over ten years ago when he first moved to Hong Kong—and believe me, back then he was not known as the "fitness guy" in any circles. I would run into him in the gym occasionally, but nothing about his physique made me raise an eyebrow.

But over the last few years I noticed a significant change in both his physicality and his overall attitude. He slimmed down significantly from when I first met him and was much more energetic. I was intrigued. We had both started off at the same point, but here I was stuck still spinning my wheels, while he had moved forward by leaps and bounds.

Out of curiosity, and ultimately frustration, I finally confronted him and asked him what his workout was like. It was then that Jay presented his *Hack Your Fitness* lifestyle program to me. At first it seemed unorthodox, but I was desperate for a solution. I was ready to take drastic measures and make a lifestyle change.

Jay offered to personally coach me through his program, and I agreed without hesitation. In truth, I wasn't interested in learning all the details and granular science behind fitness; I just wanted to be told what to do and when to do it. I just wanted the results, and I wanted them fast.

As you can guess, his program worked wonders for me and changed my life. Within just a few months of starting Jay's *Hack Your Fitness* lifestyle program, I knew that it was the solution I'd been searching for during my entire career. In just three months, I slashed twenty-one pounds of body fat and made huge gains in all my lifts. Most importantly, his system was flexible and sustainable for my extremely busy lifestyle. I carried on for a couple of more months with the program and lost another fourteen pounds for a total fat loss of thirty-five pounds, earning me a whole new physique.

Hack Your Fitness was a game changer in my life. It presents a fresh angle to the fitness industry, allowing everyday people to get into the best shape of their lives without the crazy six-day training routines.

Jay spent the past fifteen years of his life tirelessly researching and testing various methods and systems in fitness and nutrition. Jay's book, *Hack Your Fitness*, is the culmination of all those countless hours of research distilled into a simple system that is easily adoptable by anyone at any stage of personal fitness.

This book breaks down all myths and dogmas that plague the health and fitness industry today and gives you the exact blueprint to achieve the same level of freedom in fitness that I did. It is filled with information that will teach you the simple science behind diet and nutrition and show you how to train in the most efficient and effective way possible, saving you hours a week. It's a novel approach for high achievers and busy professionals like myself who don't have the time to spend countless hours in the gym doing mundane cardio or reading fitness magazines.

As we get older, our lives only get busier. We have less time for family, less time for our careers, and less time for fitness. A few years ago, I cofounded my own racing team, Craft-Bamboo Racing. I continue to compete internationally and have gotten married to the love of my life, Amber. I still travel extensively for much of the year. Through it all, I am 100 percent in control of my nutrition and fitness. I am armed with the knowledge to face any situation that life throws my way.

As an athlete and an entrepreneur, I know firsthand that whenever you try to achieve something outside of your comfort zone, there always exists a fear of failure. But I can say with confidence that *Hack Your Fitness* is one system that will not fail you. If you follow Jay's methods to a tee, you will be successful, and that is a guarantee.

When it comes down to it, *Hack Your Fitness* shares one of the same tenants that my father instilled in me as a child, and that is to invest in yourself. Educate yourself. Learn the simple science behind nutrition and fitness. Learn how to train smart and efficiently.

This book is about freeing yourself from the shackles of fitness and taking control so you can move on to improve other aspects of your life. It's about saving time that can be spent on family and career.

If you picked up this book, it's because you've struggled with the same things I have and are searching for a solution. You're searching for freedom. This is the last fitness book your will ever have to read. It's the straightest line to success. Run and grab a copy, and start hacking your fitness today.

— DARRYL O'YOUNG, PROFESSIONAL RACE CAR DRIVER

2015 GT ASIA SERIES CHAMPION

2013 SECOND IN CLASS IN 24 HOURS OF LE MANS

THREE-TIME WINNER OF MACAU GRAND PRIX

TWO-TIME PORSCHE CARRERA CUP ASIA CHAMPION

TWO-TIME WINNER OF 12 HOURS OF BATHURST

INTRODUCTION

What we face may look insurmountable. But I learned
something from all those years of training and competing.
I learned something from all those sets and reps when I didn't
think I could lift another ounce of weight. What I learned is
that we are always stronger than we know.

— ARNOLD SCHWARZENEGGER

I never thought the turning point of my fitness journey
would be a gut-punch comment from my wife as I prepared
to take a shower. Yet as she gazed upon the upper body I
had spent years crafting, something compelled her to fling
this particular dagger my way:

"For someone who works out all the time, you're actually not that jacked."

Her shot hit me right where my six-pack should have been, and that was the problem. I was known as the "fitness guy" within my social circle because I'd spent years educating myself on various methods of diet and exercise. Despite my steadfast commitment, I knew deep down that I hadn't achieved the body I actually wanted.

My wife's comment didn't just sting because it came from someone who loved me and showed her support for my goals by prepping all my meals over the years. It stung because she was right. Her delivery could've been better, but her message was spot on.

Did I realize that right away? Of course not. I was in the shower just fuming about this comment from my wife, who is blessed to be what I call a "genetic freak." She's naturally lean, can eat whatever she wants, and doesn't have to work out. "It's not fair," I grumbled to myself as the hot water streamed down my face. "I work my ass off to have a body like hers. What the hell does she know about fitness anyway? How could she say that to me?"

I'm not proud of my feelings in the shower that day.

As the hours went by, her comment kept eating away at me until I stepped back and asked myself, "Why is this bothering me so much?" That's when I realized the problem was with me, not with what she said. As always, she was right.

A cutting truth like that is not easy to hear when you're working out six days a week, doing a shit ton of cardio, and eating "clean" in order to achieve single-digit body fat. I wanted a six-pack so badly, and my wife knew that. In fact, I'm pretty sure that's why she made her comment in the first place—she subconsciously knew I needed a wake-up call.

Still, this realization frustrated me because I'd committed so much time and energy to getting that six-pack. I was eating six meals a day after reading Tom Venuto's book *Burn the Fat, Feed the Muscle* and learning that bodybuilders used that eating schedule to maintain their metabolism and feed their muscles. I slimmed down considerably using Tom's system in 2008, going from 183 pounds with 20 percent body fat to 165 pounds and 15 percent body fat in just three months.

I figured the final step in achieving single-digit body fat was finding the right exercise for my body type, which translated to me trying every workout under the sun: twice-a-day cardio, high-intensity interval training, P90X, Shaun

T's Insanity, SoulCycle classes, kickboxing, and CrossFit. I even tried rowing for a while. After all that sweat, my body fat still refused to budge.

Before settling on six meals a day, I'd also tried different diets: Atkins low-carb, Tim Ferriss's slow carb diet, paleo—you name it, I gave it a whirl at some point. The only thing those diets made me realize was how much I hated dieting.

For the life of me, I couldn't figure out what I was missing. I had tried every answer in the book, and none of them got me over the hump and into the promised land of single-digit body fat. Was there some hidden secret I had yet to stumble upon?

It turns out there was no secret I was missing, no magic formula awaiting me on the other side of a mirror in my local gym. I had everything I needed after years of surveying the landscape and acquiring a vast knowledge of nutrition and exercise. My problem was simply not putting the pieces together in the right order.

I had a syntax error.

In the world of computer programming, a syntax error results from a character or string being placed incorrectly in a command and causing a failure in execution.

It's no different than what my wife used to do at bars before we were married. When a guy would approach her and ask for her number, and she didn't really want to give it to him, she would give her number but switch the last two digits. The number looked legit, and she could recite it easily, but when the guy would call, he wouldn't get through.

That's the idea of syntax error. You have all the right numbers but in the wrong sequence. You don't get through. Most people who want to be fit can easily learn about fitness now with a quick Google search, some YouTube videos, and a couple of Bodybuilding.com articles. It's not hard to acquire the information you need when you want something as bad as I wanted a six-pack.

But, as Tony Robbins says, "What you know doesn't mean shit." It's getting the right combination that counts.

Uncovering this truth in 2014 was a paradigm shift for me. I'd spent fifteen years dialing the wrong sequence and nearly gave up. When I figured out the right sequence—the one I'm going to teach you in this book—my whole life changed. With the correct syntax, it took me just three months to reach single-digit body fat and achieve my six-pack.

That's the reason I wrote this book. I'm not a fitness professional, nor do I have any fancy degrees or certifications hanging on my wall. I'm simply an everyday desk jockey who experienced the same kind of pain I know a lot of you are dealing with today. I've been where you are and suffered through all the exhausting workouts, unending meal prep, and constant sacrifices that are meant to improve your level of fitness but only leave you short of your true goals.

Those shitty days are over, my friend.

MINIMUM EFFECTIVE FITNESS PROTOCOL

Time is an equal opportunity employer. Each human being has exactly the same number of hours and minutes every day. Rich people can't buy more hours. Scientists can't invent new minutes. You can't save time to spend it on another day.

— DENIS WAITLEY

I'm thirty-seven years old with two kids, which means I don't have time to spend hours working on my fitness each week. My goals have changed, as well. When I was younger, I wanted to look like Arnold Schwarzenegger. I think all guys go through that phase where they want to be able to bench X amount so they can look like a *Men's Health* model.

Now I just care about being lean. When you get lean, your body looks better visually and you actually look bigger even though you've trimmed down. Because my life is so busy with kids and work, I wanted to get lean in the shortest amount of time possible.

That's where the idea of a "minimum effective fitness protocol" (MEFP) originated. If you're strapped for time and want a complete nutrition and fitness system that is highly efficient, this is the solution you've been searching for.

MEFP is an adaptation of the "minimum effective dose" (MED) that I first read about in Tim Ferriss's book *The 4-Hour Body*. As Tim explains, MED is "the smallest dose that will produce a desired outcome... Anything beyond the MED is wasteful. To boil water, the MED is 212°F (100°C) at standard air pressure. Boiled is boiled. Higher temperatures will not make it 'more boiled.' Higher temperatures just consume more resources that could be used for something else more productive."

My program is the Minimum Effective Fitness Protocol for high achievers like you and I who want maximum results from minimum time and effort. I'm giving you the straightest line between where you are now and the results you seek: single-digit body fat and six-pack abs for life.

If fitness is a priority in your life but you've never achieved the body fat level you want, or haven't gotten as lean as you'd like, *Hack Your Fitness* is the last fitness book you'll ever need to read. The same goes for people who are busy with a family or have demanding careers and can't devote an hour a day to working out.

With my system, you don't need that much time, because *Hack Your Fitness* optimizes this area of your life. Don't misunderstand me. You're going to work your ass off on this program, but in terms of hours spent each week on diet and exercise, the commitment is minimal.

I don't think twice about fitness anymore. I give it forty-five minutes, three times a week, and then I check it off my list. I cherish the extra time I have now that I'm not combing through fitness magazines, and I love saving money since I'm not eating six times a day or bouncing from one diet or exercise DVD to the next looking for answers.

I'm going to be very honest with you. *Hack Your Fitness* is not one of these Fitness 101 books where I examine every aspect of nutrition and exercise in detail. Remember, I'm trying to save you time here.

Some people might have different fitness goals than those I've outlined in this book, and that's okay. If your immediate goal is to look like Arnold Schwarzenegger, you're better off looking elsewhere for a book to get you there. Or if you want to compete in a marathon or a triathlon, or if you're into cycling, I'm sad to say that *Hack Your Fitness* does not include any cardio whatsoever.

Hack Your Fitness is a lifestyle solution that streamlines your fitness to require the minimum amount of your precious time as possible. At times, I too enjoy the social aspect of working out like anyone else, but my program is not, "Let's go to the gym and chitchat around the water cooler and get a set in." You go in, get your shit done, and get out. I don't even go to the gym anymore, since I have a squat rack at home. That's all you need for this program.

Finally, I have to add the disclaimer that, while I've seen amazing results from women using *Hack Your Fitness*, pregnant women should not attempt this program, because it's so physically demanding. Nor should women who are still breastfeeding postpartum, since they should not be in a twelve-week caloric restriction. (Newborns need their calories!) When in doubt, always consult with your physician before beginning a rigorous exercise program.

I pride myself on having an honest and transparent approach to fitness, which is sadly something I can't say for all programs out there, or for the fitness industry in general.

SMOKE AND MIRRORS

We live in a world that seems increasingly beyond our control.
The less we attempt, the less chance of failure.

— ROBERT GREENE

There's a saying: "Don't ask a barber if you need a haircut."

Unfortunately, that's the state of fitness as I see it right now. Don't ask a trainer if you need to exercise more, or question a supplement specialist about the need for his or her product.

The fitness industry has transformed over the past few decades into a large marketing monster that preys on human insecurities and desires. For all the trainers out there, only a small number actually train with integrity, purpose, and the right intent. The rest are symptomatic of an industry that's more concerned with obtaining your money than giving you results.

How many of these deceptions and half-truths have you seen recently?

"Eat six meals a day or your metabolism will slow down!"

"Without this miracle supplement or shake, your workouts won't have the full effect!"

"Our exercise program gives you the ONLY comprehensive workout in the world!"

Each of these claims disguises its intention to sell you something. If companies were honest and said you could achieve the body you want with no supplements, they'd be wiping out a multibillion-dollar industry. We all know that's not going to happen.

You can't escape this profit-driven mind-set. Think about the last fitness magazine you picked up. Chances are you saw one page of advertisements for every page of content, or you got four pages into what you thought was a great article, but at the end you found out it was actually a sponsored "advertorial" prepared by a company trying to sell you a fitness program or supplement.

One of the benefits of my program is not having to waste your time or money on these magazines anymore. Since reading Venuto's book in 2008, I've moved away from these inaccurate, money-sucking publications and used legitimate resources such as the National Institute of Health and scholarly articles in respected peer-reviewed publications.

You no longer have to wade around in the vast pool of misinformation that's out there. With all the money flying around in the health and fitness industry, the landscape is littered with pitfalls you need to avoid. Flip through the wrong magazine or stumble upon an inaccurate website, and you can end up misinformed or suffering from a syntax error.

As we get older, we become more reluctant to reconsider something that's been ingrained in our minds for years. These so-called truths are known as invisible scripts and have a much greater impact on our actions than we realize. Think about the food pyramid we all learned about in school. The Department of Agriculture introduced that guide in 1992, and some people still follow it religiously despite its being replaced in 2011 with the MyPlate guide.

You need an open but skeptical mind if you're going to survive on your own amid the sea of nutrition and exercise information that's out there. Once you accept a piece of information as fact, it's extremely difficult to break through that "pillar of truth" even if it's been proven wrong by updated research and information.

If avoiding these pitfalls sounds too stressful for you, you've come to the right place. In *Hack Your Fitness*, I'm going to give you all the information you need to accomplish your goals so you never have to worry about diet or exercise research again.

You've got better things to do with your time and money!

SIMPLE BUT NOT EASY

If you don't make time for exercise, you'll probably have to make time for illness.

— ROBIN SHARMA

Look, I get it—working out isn't necessarily fun. I can't tell you the last morning I woke up excited to exercise that day. I wish we lived in a world where everyone was blessed with fast metabolisms and rock-hard abs. (I'm not sure what this book would be about in that alternate reality, but I'd gladly make that trade!)

The simple yet difficult-to-swallow fact is that fitness is an integral part of living a healthy life. We all know this, but because of our increasingly busy lives, we have a hard time making our fitness a priority. I feel your pain, and that's why I'm providing you with the quickest, most efficient way to achieve and maintain single-digit body fat for the rest of your life. Just give me twelve weeks of your life, and I can all but guarantee that you'll see significant results.

But maybe your guard is still up. You've seen these kinds of promises before in other fitness books, and they've all turned out to be empty. I get it. Like I said, you should approach everything in this industry with an open but skeptical mind.

Here's where my program differs from those you've tried in the past: This is not a "get fit quick" scheme. It's also not focused on "biohacking" your body like *The Tim Ferriss Experiment*. Biohacking is trendy right now, but many of the results are unproven. *Hack Your Fitness* gives you proven results by teaching you the simple science behind fitness and nutrition.

I'm telling you right now that *Hack Your Fitness* is simple, but it's not easy. If you're looking for easy, I'm here to tell you that option doesn't exist. There is no way short of liposuction to get lean overnight, no fitness lottery you can hope to win.

These next twelve weeks are going to be difficult. This process takes a lot of mental discipline and fortitude. You need willpower and patience to get through *Hack Your Fitness*.

But if you follow this protocol to the letter for twelve weeks, you're going to transform your body into a lean machine. I have compressed the time you need to spend on fitness because I remember the misery of working out six days a week, doing twice-a-day cardio, virtually killing myself trying to get lean. I got nowhere near my goals, and it frustrated the hell out of me.

You don't have to go through what I did in order to transform your body. Whatever methods you've learned for getting lean, this is a simpler way that involves less time.

Again, it's simple, but it's not easy. *Hack Your Fitness* is as much a mental fitness program as it is a physical fitness program. When people think about health and fitness, their minds jump straight to working out and the tactics they need to fix their bad habits.

This program is much more of a mental challenge. You have to clean up your diet by counting your calories and tracking your macros. You have to be open to the concept of skipping breakfast as part of intermittent fasting. The gym is not going to be your biggest challenge. Breakfast meetings are going to be your stumbling blocks. Thanksgiving is now the enemy.

Remember: You can't outwork a bad diet.

Let's talk about the workouts for a minute. When we're in the gym, we're giving max effort on our compound lifts and pushing ourselves to the point of near failure. We're not going to be on the bike checking Facebook for forty-five minutes. If you come in and give it everything you have, you get to walk out and be done for the day. It's not easy, but it's that simple.

By following *Hack Your Fitness*, you're going to have a better shot at maintaining the body you achieve through this program. Our body has certain set points, and when you get down to a set point and maintain that for a while, it's easier to get back to that point if you have a relapse.

I achieved my first set point back in 2008 when I went from 183 down to 165 pounds. For the next few years, if I had a binge weekend where I shot up to 170, it was no big deal for me to get back down to 165. I maintained that weight long enough that it became my floor.

My set point is much lower now after using this system for the past two years. My new weight is 153 pounds with 8 percent body fat. When my wife and I enjoyed a weekend in Tokyo recently—our first getaway from the kids in about three years—I went nuts. I ate and drank like I'd just been released from prison, and when we got back to Hong Kong, I weighed 160 pounds.

Within forty-eight hours, my weight had already gone back down to 154. Amazing.

These next twelve weeks are going to change the rest of your life. You're going to see gains like you've never seen before and easily maintain those gains going forward. This program isn't one of those six-week cuts you do before vacation where you rebound miserably afterward. When you get down, my maintenance protocol will keep you there.

A lifetime of results demands a lifestyle change, and that's what *Hack Your Fitness* teaches you. Most people might see a diet as a temporary thing, but your diet is really the way you eat your food on a regular basis, for life. If needed, this book will change your mind-set about eating. Rest assured, once you've finished the program, there's more flexibility on what you can eat. I'm not going to take away fried chicken or pizza from you forever.

I'd rather teach you to fish than give you a fish, so I've designed this protocol with one purpose in mind: to empower you to change your life for the better. But that means you have to look yourself in the mirror and say, "I'm ready to make a change in my life."

I can't be there every single time to look over your shoulder when you're tracking your macros, or offer a critique on your squatting technique. Your fitness destiny is in your hands.

Hack Your Fitness is something you'll do for the next twelve weeks, and once you see the results, you'll want to keep hacking for the rest of your live. It's that simple, and it's that straightforward.

KEY TAKEAWAYS

◯ When it comes to fitness, it's not what you know but applying it in the right order that counts. A syntax error, or doing things in the wrong order, leads to fitness frustration.

◯ If you're strapped for time, you need the Minimum Effective Fitness Protocol (MEFP). This is the straightest line between where you are now and six-pack abs and single-digit body fat.

◯ The fitness industry is more concerned with taking your money than giving you honest exercise or diet advice. *Hack Your Fitness* allows you to avoid the cesspool of fitness misinformation that's out there.

◯ This book is not a "get fit quick" scheme. Short of liposuction, overnight weight loss is not possible. Lasting results require patience.

◯ True fitness is more of a mental challenge than a physical one because you need the willpower to change your diet in addition to working out.

◯ *Hack Your Fitness* allows you to maintain your results long-term if you understand that a lifetime of results demands a lifestyle change.

ACTION STEPS

🧍 Forget what you *think* you know about fitness and nutrition.

🧍 Commit to making a lifestyle change that will radically improve your life.

🧍 Start mentally preparing yourself for a challenging next 12 weeks.

—

PART ONE

MIND OVER MATTER

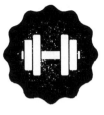

CHAPTER 1

THE PSYCHOLOGY OF FITNESS

Next to physical survival, the greatest need of a human being is psychological survival—to be understood, affirmed, validated and appreciated.

— STEVEN COVEY

Before we dive into the tactics of diet and exercise, I want to have an honest moment of reflection about why human beings want to get fit. To do that, let's take a look back at my fitness journey and examine how my motivation evolved over the years.

When a person begins working out, his or her decision is

usually the result of a certain trigger. It might be a New Year's resolution, a pair of pants that are too tight, or perhaps even a passing comment very much like the one my wife gave me. Whatever the case, that trigger makes this person want to get serious about fitness.

When I started working out in 2001, I didn't know my trigger. I was working on Wall Street at the time, and when I saw my colleagues going to the gym after work or overheard them talking about their workouts, I figured I should probably start working out, too.

The only problem was I had no idea what I was doing. Fitness was a career accessory, not a building block for my life. If I didn't have time to work out, I quickly forgave myself for not having the energy after sixty-hour work weeks and nights spent out entertaining clients. If I did make time, I'd cherry-pick workouts I saw in the latest issue of *Men's Health* and would try those until I got tired of them. I never tracked my gains or worried about proper nutrition.

I look back on those days and shudder at my own ignorance. I did that useless song and dance from 2001 to 2005 while I lived in New York and made zero progress.

In fact, I actually got fatter.

I decided in 2006 that I would try working out in order to be healthy. That's a good motivation, right? I lit my fire with that fuel for a while, and the flame only flickered. Health was part of the answer, but it wasn't my end trigger. I had to keep looking.

A few years later, I decided that my new motivation would be to get stronger. I wanted to be able to lift more weight at the gym than anyone else my size. Surely this one would stick, I figured. Who doesn't want to be strong? Yet again, my motivation flickered and faded like a wind-blown flame. Getting stronger, like being healthier, was merely another step toward figuring out my true trigger.

I decided I should sit back and let true motivation find me...and find me, it did. The answer was revealed in my reflection—pants that were too tight and a gut that always protruded when I wore dress shirts. "This is horrible," I said to myself. "I look like shit!"

In this very vain, superficial moment of honesty, I discovered my bottom-line reason for working out: I wanted to look good. Like that model on the cover of *Men's Health*, I wanted to be lean with six-pack abs and a shredded physique. I knew that people tended to judge others based on their outward appearance, and I didn't want someone's first impression of me to be, "Get a load of this fat-ass with the tight pants and the beer gut."

My reasoning was definitely superficial. But can you deny that society treats good-looking people better than it treats bad-looking people? Human beings are vain like that. They want to look good and surround themselves with others who look good, too.

I told you that *Hack Your Fitness* is an honest program, and quite honestly, fitness has always been about vanity to me. Health is a secondary concern. Looking good is the trigger that gets me out of bed three times a week and into my home gym. Being healthy is a nice side benefit of fitness, but I think if you're honest with yourself, you'll find that your motivation closely resembles mine. There is nothing wrong with wanting to look good, which means there is nothing wrong with admitting your vanity and owning it.

If you're standing with me and proudly saying you want to look good, that's going to be our fitness goal. If your honest moment of introspection reveals a different motivation, that's totally fine! I believe most people are fueled by vanity, but there are those with more noble intentions. It only matters that you have a goal that carries some sort of emotional investment. This is the only way you will find success in this program, and that's why I wanted to strip away the bullshit and get to the heart of why you picked up this book.

Now that we understand why we want to get fit, let's examine some of the reasons people come up short with their fitness goals so we can avoid falling into those traps.

REFRAME YOUR LIFESTYLE

A wise man will be master of his mind, a fool will be its slave.

— PUBLILIUS SYRUS

I mentioned in the introduction how many people share the mentality that diets are temporary and not a lifestyle change. "How long is your diet?" We hear this question asked all the time, and the answer is usually something like, "I'm off carbs this month."

There is no bigger impediment to maintaining your desired level of fitness than this "pick it up and put it down" mindset. Results simply don't last when you drop a diet and go back to eating like you did before. Without a focus on maintenance and longevity, you better believe those love handles will be coming back with a vengeance.

The program found in this book lasts twelve weeks, but the *Hack Your Fitness* lifestyle is something you'll adopt for the rest of your life. If you're not eating the right food, I'm going to educate you on what foods you should be eating. When someone asks how your diet is going, you'll describe to them what your way of eating is like, for life. Proper nutrition doesn't adhere to a timeframe, nor does it take a vacation during the summer or around the holidays.

Fortunately for you, we live in an age where it's actually cool to be fit. In the 1960s, every nuclear family was eating mayonnaise sandwiches and drinking colas made with real sugar. Nobody gave a shit about fitness except your crazy uncle, and his idea of a weight-loss plan was to strap a tire around his waist and sweat away the pounds.

If you can wrap your mind around the idea of this program as a lifestyle change, you'll find that your chances of success are much higher now that our lives are so intertwined with the Internet. I lived in New York a decade ago, and fitness hadn't burst on the scene quite like it has now, thanks to the Internet. Back in the day it was much easier to succumb to social pressure if you were trying to eat healthy or had cut out drinking. Now there are groups you can join that support you and message boards filled with encouragement.

Social media and smartphones have changed the fitness world forever with the sheer volume of pictures being posted online of ourselves every day. Between Instagram, Snapchat, and our universal acceptance of selfies, there now exists a social pressure not to have the reaction to our photos be, "Wow, so and so has put on weight."

Dislike. Unfavorite. Thumbs down emoji.

Nobody wants to elicit that kind of silent response when they post a photo. People are vain, and they want to look good in the photos they send out (#nofilter). Getting to that point is simply a matter of adapting the right psychology for a commitment to fitness.

Not everyone is capable of this mind-set shift. But those who can handle such change will find that the benefits of fitness extend beyond your body to your mind and your life.

THE POWER OF EXERCISE

The single most powerful investment we could ever make in life is investment in ourselves.

— STEVEN COVEY

Exercise is about so much more than the physical result you get from it. I didn't realize this until I had a lengthy phone call with Dr. John Ratey after reading his book *Spark* and encountered his body of research that shows a connection between physicality and a person's cognitive function. Six-pack abs might be what lights my fire, but *Spark* went a long way toward affirming my mission.

Internationally recognized as an expert in neuropsychiatry,

Ratey scientifically proves in this book that when you exercise, you work more nerve cells in your brain than during any other human activity. If you think of your brain as a muscle, he argues, then it stands to reason that your brain will atrophy just like other muscles if you don't exercise. That's why you see cognitive decline as people get older and don't exercise their bodies (and thus their minds) as frequently.

His thesis is that you can directly combat this decline through exercise. In essence, exercise makes you smarter and directly affects your future potential for success.

Tony Robbins likes to say that success leaves clues. When he studies the habits of successful people, which habit do you think Robbins sees more than any other? You guessed it: a commitment to fitness. President Obama, like a lot of presidents, works out often and in the mornings. Mark Cuban gets in at least an hour of cardio a day. Oprah is a fan of yoga, and even Warren Buffett works out so he can continue drinking Coca-Cola.

Fitness is what is called a keystone habit in that it will trigger change in many other areas of your life. For example, an exercise routine can help you cut out bad habits such as smoking. When you begin to see your body change due to exercise, you're automatically going to want to eat better so as not to undo all that hard work. Busy entrepreneurs swear by fitness as their number-one daily productivity hack. Start your morning with exercise, and you'll be more productive and better organized for the rest of your day.

The benefits to your body don't end with your abs. When you're leaner and stronger, you just operate better as a human being. You can lift a suitcase easier because you've spent time deadlifting in the gym.

You still might throw your back out, but the chances go down significantly!

There are many health benefits that come with lower body fat. I remember taking a full physical examination before I started this program where the doctor told me I was okay except for my cholesterol, which was a bit high. A year later, when I went back for my annual physical, my cholesterol had come way down. That's not a coincidence.

It's not an exaggeration to say that fitness causes every area of your life to improve. The development of new habits is one change you'll find essential to *Hack Your Fitness*.

AUTOMATE YOUR LIFE WITH HABITS

We are what we repeatedly do. Excellence then is not an act, but a habit.

— ARISTOTLE

In his book *Habit Stacking*, author S. J. Scott discusses a concept known as "cognitive load," which asserts that because we as human beings have a finite limit on our short-term memories, we must rely on our long-term memories, habits, and established procedures to do pretty much anything.

We practice habits every day. Brushing your teeth, for instance, is something you probably do every morning without thinking. It's not a chore to brush your teeth, because the act requires no additional cognitive effort. It's simply something you do. Scott says that 40 percent of actions we perform each day aren't actually decisions but habits. You don't think, "I need to brush my teeth." It's an automatic behavior.

It is crucial to understand that habits are an integral part of fitness because they remove decision making from the equation. The human brain is efficient and is constantly looking for ways to save effort, and because of this it will automatically turn almost any routine into a habit. Think about how powerful that notion is if you're struggling to make time for workouts or trying to resist bad foods. Once you make the conscious choice and practice it enough times to make it routine, your brain will take over from there and automatically turn it into a habit!

If 40 percent of our life is automated, we should strive to make fitness part of that 40 percent by adding it to our daily habits. Experts in behavior modification say it takes about twenty-eight days to form a new habit. The good news is that *Hack Your Fitness* is a twelve-week program, and I guarantee that by the end, fitness will be part of the 40 percent of your life that is automated.

I started working out in the morning in 2003, long before I got serious about fitness. I was definitely not a morning person (I don't think anyone actually is), but I did it long enough that my brain automated the process and I stopped dreading those wake-up calls. Early workouts are part of my daily routine just like brushing my teeth. In fact, on workout days when I miss a workout, I feel as if I didn't brush my teeth. My whole day is thrown off.

I like early morning workouts because they leave no room for excuses. When most people start a fitness program, it's not laziness or a lack of motivation that derails them. It's life. Life simply gets in the way. Maybe the quick happy hour drink with your boss somehow becomes ten, or you have a family member's birthday dinner to attend, or your best friend is visiting from out of town. Whatever it is, you can't always control how you spend your time after work, but you can always wake up an hour earlier to work out in the morning.

When I made the switch, I found motivation in the fact that if I accomplished nothing else the rest of the day, at least I got my workout in. As I went along, I found that by the time I got to work, I was so charged up, thanks to my workout, that my mind was already firing on all cylinders. Adopting that simple habit totally changed my life.

Your willpower to work out is like a fuel tank. As the day goes on, your job and other responsibilities will drain that fuel tank, and if you leave your workout until after you finish your day job, you might not have the motivation left to follow through on that commitment.

Early workouts allow you to jump-start your day and make fitness a priority. You'll find that life rarely gets in the way when you wake up early (and I say that as the parent of two young girls). I know that waking up early sucks. The good news is that it gets easier every time you wake up because your brain is working hard to automate that habit.

You're also instilling your life with discipline, another essential part of *Hack Your Fitness.*

COMPLIMENTS AND CANDY BARS COME FROM DISCIPLINE

Never give up what you want the most for what you want today.

— NEAL A. MAXWELL

I don't want you to give up your goal of that shredded six-pack for what you want today, whether it's an extra hour of sleep, a slice of pizza, or drinks after work.

Temporary satisfaction is not worth the setbacks caused by indulgence.

Discipline is difficult to wrangle at first, but it's too important to this program for you not to fight that battle with yourself. You can train yourself to be more disciplined just like you can train to strengthen your muscles. Because discipline is also a habit, it gets easier the longer you practice it, and you'll have plenty of opportunities to practice discipline in this program.

Going to the gym, counting calories, tracking your macros, and intermittent fasting all require a high level of discipline. When you train yourself to stick with this program and block out those temporary distractions, your life is going to improve dramatically.

But let's face it, we aren't all robots here. If you're struggling with discipline, or despairing because your new six-pack seems so far away, I find it helps to set up some rewards for yourself along the way. It's difficult to have only one big, end reward and keep working at it for twelve weeks, because quite frankly we all crave occasional rewards for our hard work along the way. These little victories validate our efforts and refuel our motivation tank.

The *Hack Your Fitness* program provides three kinds of rewards: physical, psychological, and emotional. The physical reward comes in the form of calorie cycling. Basically, on workout days, you get to eat more calories than on rest days. I actually encourage you after your workout to include a cheat element in your first meal, whether it's something sweet or some particular food you like.

You'll still need to track this item, but cheat elements are better for long-term sustainability of the program than just going in cold turkey from the start.

My cheat element is a candy bar. It's strange—back when I was spinning my wheels with fitness, I didn't eat sweets even though I loved them. Now that I've found success with my program, that success includes a candy bar, which is the opposite of most people's first instinct.

This isn't just any candy bar, mind you. It's a Quest bar, made by the powerhouse food company Quest Nutrition. Quest was cofounded by Tom Bilyeu, who is one of the smartest entrepreneurs I've ever met. In just six years he turned a fledgling start-up in a declining market into a $1 billion "unicorn" company. How did he manage to do this? In a recent phone conversation I had with him, he told me their secret to success in such a crowded market was to create a product that people would choose first by taste, which also happened to be good for them. This approach is fundamentally opposite to what every other nutrition company does, and it has clearly paid off. There's hardly a nutrition store in the world now that doesn't carry their products.

Their motto is "#CheatClean," which I love because it definitely feels as if you're cheating with flavors like cookies and cream, s'mores, double chocolate chunk, and white chocolate raspberry. I'm salivating thinking about them. Most protein bars are basically just candy bars, which is why I don't recommend eating them. (We'll talk about this later in the chapter on meal planning and nutrition). Quest Bars are an exception because the ingredients are wholesome—and they taste amazing.

So that's my physical reward. Yours will likely look different, but make sure it's something like Quest Bars that allows you to "cheat clean" and stay on track with your diet.

The second kind of reward, psychological, comes from tracking your workouts. When it comes to fitness, there are few things that feel better than successfully hitting that last rep of your work set. Tracking every lift you do creates such a big sense of accomplishment when you're able to see your forward progress week after week. You're not going to know if you don't track it, though. Beyond being key to your success with *Hack Your Fitness* and the source of your psychological reward, tracking will motivate you to rebound if you have a bad workout or a bad week.

The ultimate emotional reward comes when you reach your end goal. Along the way, you'll feel an incredible sense of pride and accomplishment when people you haven't seen in a while say to you, "Have you lost a lot of weight? You look amazing!" This social affirmation makes you feel great because you put in the work and people are finally noticing.

You have to appreciate moments like these and celebrate the minor victories in order to reach the finish line. I feel bad for people who don't savor these rewards. They just see everything as the expected outcome of their efforts. It's all so...sterile.

Count your weekly accomplishments as rewards, and celebrate them wholeheartedly. If you reframe your progress like this, these milestones will inspire you along the way.

Arnold Schwarzenegger also has some ideas when it comes to inspiration.

SEEING IS BELIEVING

We all have great inner power. The power is self-faith. There's really an attitude to winning. You have to see yourself winning before you win. You have to be hungry. You have to want to conquer.

— ARNOLD SCHWARZENEGGER

Schwarzenegger is one of my fitness heroes, and he talks about how his success in bodybuilding started with this vision he had of being crowned Mr. Olympia. He created a vivid mental image of himself on stage flexing with the crowd in front of him. He could feel the weight of both the medal around his neck and the trophy wrapped in his fingers.

Every time he faced challenges or lacked motivation, Schwarzenegger would go back to that mental image, and it would power him through the day. That's how powerful the imagery was.

Michael Phelps is another athlete who visualized his success long before he achieved it. When Phelps was younger, his swimming coach Bob Bowman would tell him to visualize the perfect race ending with Phelps's victory. Bowman called it "the videotape."

"Play the videotape first thing when you wake up," he told Phelps, and his pupil did just that. Over and over he'd play out this perfect race in his mind, and each time it ended with victory. Before bed, he'd fire the videotape up again and fall asleep with it playing in his mind.

Bowman knew what he was doing. By the time he swam in the Olympics, Phelps's victory was all but assured. The videotape was so ingrained in his mind that his body simply followed along with the moves he'd seen a thousand times before.

Both athletes demonstrate the power of imagery and visualization that is necessary to reach your goals. They had a "north star" they could reference any time they needed a reminder of where they were headed. I don't think they could have reached the pinnacle of their respective fields without it, and that's why I think it's crucial for people who jump into fitness to do so with a clear goal in mind. You need your own videotape.

It's not enough just to say you want single-digit body fat. I want you to visualize yourself with that six-pack. Take a picture of yourself, cut the head off, and put it on that fitness model's body. Make your mental videotape a pool party where you walk out with your shirt off and heads turn. That moment is your north star. It will get you through the ups and downs.

Visualization fosters a strong emotional investment in your goal. The road ahead of you is long and filled with distractions trying to knock you off course, but if you constantly replay that mental image in your mind, you're not going to give up very easily.

Once you are fully invested emotionally, your mental framework actually shifts. Schwarzenegger talks about this as well, that when you have that goal so strongly ingrained in your mind, the script will flip when you're facing day-to-day challenges. Resisting sweets is no longer a burden. Laziness ceases to be a stumbling block. Rather, these challenges become *opportunities* for you to achieve your goal, each obstacle bringing you one step closer to success. Aggravation becomes determination.

Having that visual goal really made a difference for me. For the longest time, I was one of those people who wanted to skip the mental side of things and jump straight into tactics.

It wasn't until I fell in love with the climb that I embraced the process completely. I never would have made it without picturing my ideal body at the start of each new day.

I played the videotape in my head and willed myself to make it manifest in my life. Without patience and mental fortitude, I never would've made it through twelve weeks.

Like I said, you don't get shredded overnight. Remember, you are undoing *years* of poor nutrition and inefficient exercise here. There is no lottery you can win to get lean. Results require time, and time requires resilience. You must be mentally sharp. When you embrace both sides of this endeavor—physical and mental—and possess an emotional investment tied to a strong visual goal, you're ready to take the next step.

KEY TAKEAWAYS

- ◉ Your motivation for fitness won't last unless you find your trigger—that deep emotional truth that explains why you *really* want to get fit.
- ◉ Proper nutrition is a way of eating for life, not a diet you pick up and put down.
- ◉ Dr. John Ratey showed in his book *Spark* that exercise doesn't just give you bigger muscles or a leaner physique—it also improves cognitive function.
- ◉ Fitness is a keystone habit that will trigger positive change in other areas of your life. For example, you'll stop smoking, start eating

better, and see an increase in your productivity.

○ Habits are essential to fitness because they remove the decision making from the equation. With habits, you just do; you don't think. Therefore, your goal should be to instill exercise as a new habit in your life through repeated practice.

○ Working out in the morning jump-starts your day and eliminates the excuses you might have for skipping your workout after your day job is finished.

○ Your motivational fuel tank drains throughout the day, diminishing your desire to work out as the day goes on.

○ One key to sticking with *Hack Your Fitness* for twelve weeks is setting up physical, psychological, and emotional rewards for yourself along the way.

○ You need to visualize your success in order to achieve your fitness goals. When times get tough and you want to quit, you can call on that "videotape" in your head to help you push through.

ACTION STEPS

👥 Find your trigger for fitness that can serve as unwavering motivation. You can do this by stripping away the BS and honestly answering the question: "Why do I want to get fit?"

👥 Open yourself up to the possibility of working out in the morning. Your best chance at installing fitness as a habit in your life is to get it done first thing in the morning on workout days.

👥 Find a cheat item (such as Quest Nutrition bars) that can serve as a physical reward on workout days.

👥 Create your own mental videotape, and get ready to use it.

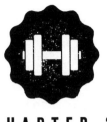

CHAPTER 2

BUILD A FITNESS FOUNDATION ON ROCK, NOT SAND

Effort for the sake of effort is as foolish a tradition as paying dues.

— SHANE SNOW

Years before my wife's comment and the shower of shame, I experienced my first fitness wake-up call at a Hong Kong gym with my brother. It was 2006 when he said something that I still carry around with me to this day:

"It seems like working out is not really a priority for you."

Ouch. Another shot from a family member that hit me right in my gut.

I was immediately defensive, firing back: "You don't understand. My job is really important to me, and I don't always have time to work out. I try to find time on the weekends or after work, but I usually have to go out and entertain clients."

Surely he could understand how busy I was and empathize with my struggle to carve out time for fitness. I was working on Wall Street for crying out loud!

He showed me no mercy, replying, "If it was a priority for you, you'd figure out how to fit it in your schedule." Now I was indignant. "Seriously, Dan, you don't understand," I shot back. "My job is really stressful. You have no right to judge my commitment to fitness."

We actually got into a tiff right there in the gym and shouted back and forth at each other. I'm not proud of what happened, but like most dudes, we got over it before the workout ended. Everything seemed fine. I didn't know it then, but his comment planted a seed in my head that would bear fruit years down the road. That day, I just shrugged it off.

For the next couple years, I kept going with what I was

doing. Fitness was just something I would sprinkle into my routine whenever I came up for air between work functions.

All that changed in 2008 when the company I was working for, Bear Stearns, went under because of the global financial crisis. And just like that, I and all my coworkers were laid off. With no idea of what to do next, I recognized that now was my opportunity to commit fully to fitness. My excuses were gone. If I didn't do it now, I knew I never would.

It took two years, but the seed my brother had planted finally blossomed.

I set to work trying to figure out where I was going wrong with fitness. That's when I first read *Burn the Fat, Feed the Muscle*. Venuto's book was actually my first attempt at trying to educate myself on the nutrition side of things. Prior to that point, I'd only focused on the tactics of working out and what I could do in the gym to beat this slow metabolism I thought I had. My knowledge of nutrition was essentially "calories in, calories out."

I thought I could outwork my poor diet by simply burning more calories than I consumed. After all, it was basic math, right? For the first period of my fitness life, that was my only belief.

Burn the Fat, Feed the Muscle was a total paradigm shift for me. I realized rather quickly that I actually knew nothing about diet and nutrition. When I came to the conclusion that 85 percent of fitness is diet and only 15 percent is exercise, I saw my failures in a whole new light. By focusing totally on exercise, I was ignoring the only part of the equation that could lead to success. No wonder I gained weight while working out—I was only doing 15 percent of the work!

Once I stopped mentally kicking myself in the ass for years of willful ignorance, I dove into research on all areas of fitness. One of the first truths I uncovered dispelled a lot of my notions concerning body types and our predisposition to exercise and diet.

Body types were first defined by American psychologist William Sheldon in the 1940s. He classified every person on a sliding scale of three main body types: ectomorphs, mesomorphs, and endomorphs.

Ectomorphs are super lean and have a hard time building muscle or keeping any weight on. Stuck in the middle are mesomorphs with their stockier, more muscular build. They hold more body fat than ectomorphs but not as much as endomorphs at the other end of the scale, which are your typical chubby guys with love handles or a belly that sticks out.

Although the three categories give us a general idea of the body type of most humans, there are a ton of factors that are at play when determining how our bodies will react to fitness, including genetics, sex, hormonal balance, age, and any medical conditions you may have. The reality is that you cannot just broadly say a person with one body type has a certain type of metabolism versus another. It's not that simple.

Of course, I didn't know any of this at the time. I called my wife a genetic freak earlier, someone who can eat whatever she wants and will remain thin without exercising. She must simply be an ectomorph. I thought of myself as more of an endomorph than an ectomorph because it was easy to blame my lack of results on a slow metabolism. All those ectomorphs with their perfect proportions and six-pack abs didn't understand the struggle we endomorphs faced!

The other excuse I loved to use was the celebrity versus noncelebrity card. If only I was a celebrity and had a personal trainer and a nutritionist like Brad Pitt has, you bet your ass I'd have the body of a Greek god. Actors, celebrities, models—their job is basically to look good. It would be easy if I had the advantages they did.

Because I wasn't a genetic freak or a celebrity with millions to pour into my fitness, I just had to work harder to achieve my ideal body. This justification helped me sleep at night. Some people have a fast metabolism, I told myself, and I have a slow metabolism. Other people are celebrities, and I am not. Life's not fair, and the world is out to get me. Wah, wah, wah...

The negative feedback loop in my mind created this chip on my shoulder that only contributed to my continued wheel spinning. As I've already mentioned, using Tom Venuto's system, I actually made great progress as I went from 183 pounds and 20 percent body fat down to 165 pounds and 15 percent body fat. I was thrilled. My wife, on the other hand, was supportive but had to be annoyed with me. In addition to handling my meal prep and cooking six meals a day, she had to put up with me becoming the pickiest eater in the world.

Still, at the time it felt as if everything was working out the way I wanted.

FITNESS GROUNDHOG DAY

It is impossible for a man to learn what he thinks he already knows.

— EPICTETUS

When one of my clients organized a boat trip for me and a

few coworkers, I was ready to show off my progress. Everyone on that boat would see what cardio and countless meals had bought me.

We were out on the boat, and everyone was jumping into the water. My time had come. I took my shirt off and prepared to strut a little. One of my colleagues—who was actually overweight—was sitting nearby. He knew how much I'd sacrificed in the name of fitness. He'd seen me in the office for the last two years eating three or four of my six meals at my desk, and he knew I worked out every morning relentlessly.

I was getting ready to jump into the water when he said, "Come on, man, where's your six-pack?" I remember that comment vividly. Coming from someone who sat next to me at work and who witnessed my commitment level firsthand, his jab hit a nerve.

Once again, it hit a nerve because he called me out. It stuck with me because he was right.

But moments like these only motivated me to push myself even harder. The following summer, I managed to drop down to single-digit body fat prior to a beach vacation my wife and I took. I did this by essentially cheating the system: I cut my calorie intake for six weeks, ate super clean, didn't drink at all, and did insane cardio workouts six days a week. It worked, but I was exhausted.

After six weeks, we finally took our beach vacation, and boy, did I look great for the first day. Then, much like the trip to Tokyo I mentioned earlier, I adopted the eating and drinking habits of an inmate coming out of prison. By the end of the trip, I was back to 15 percent body fat. No sooner had I achieved the holy grail of single-digit body fat did I lose it in a heartbeat over just a few piña coladas on the beach. It was sad, but I thought this was how life would be for me. I would work my ass off to get ripped for vacation, eat a million calories on the trip, and bounce back up to where I was before.

Even the literature I was reading at the time supported this belief. Everyone from fitness professionals to bodybuilders said getting down to single-digit body fat was nearly impossible and the process would make you miserable. They said you better like bland foods because that's all you're going to eat, and if you don't like cardio, you're screwed.

You can see now why this portion of my fitness journey was miserable. I was convinced that long-term single-digit body fat was a pipe dream. If bodybuilders couldn't maintain that level after competitions, what chance did I have?

You already know what happened next: my wife stepped in to save the day.

Hack Your Fitness is the happy ending after years of frustration, false starts, and nearly giving up more times than I can remember. The time has come to kiss your syntax error good-bye and dive into the specifics of the program that's going to change your life.

NO CRIME, NO CARDIO

Everything we hear is an opinion, not a fact. Everything we see is a perspective, not the truth.

— MARCUS AURELIUS

One of the first things you should do is take an honest look at your diet. Too many people don't realize just how much a diet affects their fitness progress, so our first step is going to be education. You need to learn the Three Laws of Nutrition and understand exactly how to leverage them to be successful. Whether we like it or not, the saying, "Abs are made in the kitchen," is actually true. But I'm not just talking about eating "clean" foods all the time. It goes way beyond that, which I'll explain in detail later on. Just realize that the sooner you educate yourself and take control of your nutrition, the sooner you'll start seeing progress.

I resisted learning the truth for a long time. I was misinformed in part because the health and fitness industries are very focused on tactics. Every time you see someone who's ripped on a magazine cover, the entire issue is about his or her workout. The diet and nutrition side of the equation is ignored. These images contributed to my syntax error.

I also resisted because eating is one of the greatest joys in life. I sympathize with those who say food is their weakness. I can train myself to exercise multiple times a week, and eventually that process will become a habit. But who has time to count calories, let alone track macros? And it certainly never gets easier to resist a slice of pizza or a juicy cheeseburger. Controlling your diet is such a psychological battle.

I turned a blind eye to the holes in my diet and instead increased my cardio. That was my remedy despite the fact that I loathe cardio. Sure, after a nice cardio session you feel good. You have endorphins pumping through your body, and there's a sense of accomplishment. Cardio also takes a lot of time and it's a lot of work, so for me, cardio was always punishment. I was paying for my sins of the foods that I ate earlier, or trying to pay it forward before a big night of eating and drinking. I was trapped in this vicious circle.

Instead of getting punished, how about not committing the crime?

If you eat fast food every single day, you're going to experience diminishing returns. The satisfaction each time you eat decreases if you're allowed to eat pizza, cookies, and burgers whenever you want. After a week of eating like that, you'd be sick of it. You'd need a salad just to not feel so gross. That's just the way human beings are.

It's way easier to eat smarter, cleaner, and not deal with the punishment. A proper diet is fuel for your system and, unlike exercise, it's not optional. You have to eat, so if you can rewire your brain to eat smart, you won't have to endure cardio as penance for your sins.

With my program, you actually don't need cardio to get lean and achieve that six-pack. The diet and exercise protocols contained in this book constitute the fastest way to get lean. There are a lot of health benefits to doing cardio, but for the purposes of this book, I don't care about those benefits. Vanity is our north star.

When we talk about building a fitness foundation, it begins with an understanding that your diet will dictate your results. If you're nervous about falling off the wagon once you begin this diet, let me assure you that I've included tips in the section on maintenance for when life gets in the way. Don't worry, it happens to the best of us. Setbacks shouldn't stop you from trying. They should motivate you to try harder going forward.

You might be surprised to find that the diet section of this book is longer than the exercise section. It makes sense, though, when you remember the fitness formula: 85 percent diet, 15 percent exercise.

THE THREE LAWS OF NUTRITION

Where there is no law, there is no freedom.

— JOHN LOCKE

Let's jump right in and begin our education. When it comes to nutrition, there are only three key principles you must learn, and these principles are ranked in a hierarchy of greatest to least impact on your fitness journey. These are the three overarching principles behind the science of body recomposition that you must leverage for success. I've listed them in order of importance based on how each one will affect your progress:

1. **The Law of Energy Balance (Calories In vs. Calories Out): In order to lose weight, the amount of calories you put into your body must be less than the amount of calories you burn.**

2. The Law of Macronutrient Balance: Finding the correct balance of macronutrients (protein, carbohydrates, and fat) is the key to rapid body recomposition.

3. The Law of Food Choices: For the purposes of body recomposition, the nutritional value of food makes little difference. (Yes, really… but it's not as simple as you think.)

In the next chapter, we will begin our exploration of this diet by looking first at the Law of Energy Balance.

KEY TAKEAWAYS

- Fitness is 85 percent diet and 15 percent exercise—you can't out-work a bad diet.
- The three general body types of human beings are ectomorph (super lean), endomorph (chubbier, muscle covered by fat), and mesomorph (stockier, muscular build). This is a sliding scale.
- But there are many other factors besides body type that affect how our bodies respond to fitness. You cannot just broadly say that a person with one body type has a certain type of metabolism versus another.
- Regardless of our genetic predisposition, we have the power to move up and down the body-type scale if we so desire.
- Don't believe the lie that living with single-digit body fat is miserable. Contrary to popular belief, it's not all about bland foods and nonstop cardio.
- The saying, "Abs are made in the kitchen," is true, even if we don't like to admit it.

○ The fitness industry's obsession with exercise and tactics—at the expense of information on diet and nutrition—contributes to syntax errors.

○ Rather than paying for the dietary crimes you're committing with exercise, you can shift your eating habits so you're not committing those crimes at all.

○ You don't need cardio to get ripped.

○ Dietary setbacks will happen. *Hack Your Fitness* will teach you how to deal with them and avoid them in the future.

○ The Law of Energy Balance (Calories In vs. Calories Out), the Law of Macronutrient Balance, and the Law of Food Choices are the Three Laws of Nutrition you need to know to get ripped.

ACTION STEPS

👤 Take an honest look at your diet. Reflect on the changes you'll need to make, and begin mentally preparing to make those changes.

👤 Realize that regardless of our genetic predisposition, we have the power to move up and down the body-type scale if we so desire.

👤 Stop with the cardio. It's awful, and you don't have to do it anymore.

PART TWO

—

YOU ARE WHAT YOU EAT

CHAPTER 3

DON'T FLY BLIND: HOW TO COUNT CALORIES

To lengthen thy life, lessen thy meals.

— BENJAMIN FRANKLIN

The honest truth is that counting calories is a pain in the ass. No one likes to count calories. It's annoying to do, and it's annoying when you see someone else doing it.

I fully empathize with this. However, counting calories is an integral part of this program. Until you learn the caloric value of food items you'll be eating on this program, you're just going to have to deal with it. It's a necessary evil. You're going to be annoying with your friends when you all go out to eat, but they'll understand. They're your friends.

Within your social circle, you'll probably be the only person who counts calories, and that's okay. I'm one of the few people in my entire social circle who counts calories. I'm also the only person in my social circle with single-digit body fat. What you'll realize is that this practice separates the people who are really fit from those who aren't.

My laziness when it came to counting calories was one of the two major roadblocks I encountered in my fitness journey. The second one was my failure to track macros, which we'll talk about later. If you don't know how many calories you're eating, you have zero chance of success. It's that simple. Unless you're a genetic freak, you have to count your calories.

I'm being blunt here because the last thing I want is for you to spin your wheels like I did. Counting calories is simple, and we're going to walk through it together.

THE FIRST LAW OF NUTRITION

What goes up must come down.

— ISAAC NEWTON

The Law of Energy Balance (Calories In vs. Calories Out)

states that in order to lose weight, the amount of calories you put into your body must be less than the amount of calories you burn.

This is like fitness's version of Newton's Law of Gravity. It's the most important law of nutrition and the overarching principle that you must never forget. It's the reason why you hear about people being able to "lose weight" when eating burgers and fries for thirty days straight, and why people like me still gained weight while working out like crazy and eating "clean." This part seems pretty self-explanatory, so why is it that so many people cannot get it right?

There are two basic truths when it comes to eating:

1. **Human beings don't need to eat as much as they think they do.**
2. **Human beings consistently underestimate the number of calories they eat.**

The reason we're like this when we eat is because we follow what are called "mindless eating scripts," a term that comes from the book *Mindless Eating* by Brian Wansink. When we get hungry, our brain triggers a cue that tells us to begin our eating ritual. The mindless eating script that most of us follow is that we'll eat until the food is gone and we feel full. Once that happens, there's another trigger that turns off the eating.

For me, part of my downfall came from growing up with parents who wouldn't let me leave the table until I finished all the food on my plate. They would always say shit like, "You don't know what it's like to be hungry. There are kids in Africa who don't get to eat, so you need to finish the food on your plate." Many of you I'm sure had a similar upbringing.

Mom and Dad meant well, but they were encouraging mindless eating. To this day, whenever I'm at a restaurant and there's food left on the table, a battle begins in my head as I think, "We should really finish that." I still want to clean my plate, regardless of how full I am. I have this mentality where I feel that uneaten food is a waste, which is frustrating.

Another fun fact from *Mindless Eating* says that when people preplate their food, they eat 14 percent less. If you're at a buffet and you only eat the food you preplate, as opposed to doing family style where you share multiple larger dishes with the table, you're going to eat less.

Then there's a third study from that same book that says human beings eat for volume. Regardless of how rich or how dense the food is calorically, you're going to eat the same amount of volume until you are full. If you have a plate full of broccoli and a plate full of Skittles, and you are looking to eat two plates of food, you're going to clean both plates regardless of the fact that a plate of Skittles has roughly one hundred times the calories of a broccoli plate. That's why the "clean your plate" mentality is counterproductive to what we're trying to accomplish with *Hack Your Fitness*.

If you're a visual person, think about counting calories as a graph of your daily spending pattern. Every day you start with an allotted budget or maximum number of calories you can "spend" that day. You start with zero calories consumed, and the goal over the course of the day is to eat no more than the maximum number of calories allowed by your budget. By charting your calorie spending each day, you'll be able to see quite quickly if you've stayed within your budget or blown right through it (like eating an entire plate of Skittles). This graph keeps you accountable, and we'll talk about some tools later to help you actually chart your calories.

STRENGTH IN NUMBERS

Alone we can do so little; together we can do so much.

— HELEN KELLER

Now that we know why counting calories is important, let's crunch some numbers. I mentioned earlier that the "calories in, calories out" formula was my starting point for understanding the diet side of fitness. This formula alone didn't lead to success, because I was missing the other key components of my plan, but it's crucial to understand how foundational this concept is to the diet we're laying out here.

To recap, the first and most important Law of Nutrition says that if you eat more calories than you burn, you're going to gain weight. If you burn more calories than you eat, you're going to lose weight. The math for this cornerstone of our diet is simple.

The first step when counting calories is figuring out exactly how many you burn on a daily basis. We do this by calculating what's called your "total daily energy expenditure" (TDEE). You might also see this referred to as your daily maintenance calories. This is the number of calories you spend every day just living your life.

There are two components to TDEE, the first of which is your basal metabolic rate (BMR). If you were in a coma and didn't move at all, the number of calories your body would need to survive is your BMR. It's the baseline of your caloric intake.

There are two popular equations for determining BMR: the Harris-Benedict equation and the Katch-McArdle equation. You can use either one, but for the Katch-McArdle, you need to know roughly what your body fat percentage is to calculate it. These equations might look scary for non-math folks, but don't panic—there are online calculators where you can plug in your numbers and get your answer if you prefer that route. Just Google "BMR Calculator." It's simple. For those of you that prefer old-school pen and paper, here is the math.

Let's start with the Harris-Benedict equation, which is specific to your gender, but the easier of the two.

HARRIS-BENEDICT EQUATION

Men's BMR = 66 + (6.23 × weight in pounds) + (12.7 × height in inches) − (6.8 × age in years)

Women's BMR = 655 + (4.35 × weight in pounds) + (4.7 × height in inches) − (4.7 × age in years)

That's it!

As I just mentioned, you'll need a rough estimate of your body fat percentage for the second BMR measurement method, which is the Katch-McArdle equation. There are many ways to obtain that measurement, and we'll cover those in more detail in the chapter on macronutrients. For now, the easiest and most accurate way to measure your body fat is to use body fat calipers. You can find them for ten to twenty dollars online if you don't own a pair. You just pinch an inch of your stomach and use the caliper to measure. It's painless and reliable.

Don't bother with those fancy scales you see at the gym. They run an electric charge through your body, and how quickly it moves depends a lot on your hydration level, which changes throughout the day. The measurements they spit out are not reliable.

Once you have your body fat percentage, the Katch-McArdle equation works for both genders.

KATCH-MCARDLE EQUATION

BMR = 370 + (21.6 × LBM); where LBM = [Weight in pounds / 2.2] – [(Weight in pounds / 2.2) * body fat %]

Both of these equations should give you roughly the same number. We're not looking for pinpoint precision here, just a close estimate of your BMR, which should be within 100 calories. When you feel confident in your math, we're going to add in an activity factor, which is the second part of calculating TDEE.

Obviously if you're a marathon runner who trains every day, you're going to burn a lot more calories than if you're used to just lying on the couch. The activity factor is used to determine your level of daily physical exertion. Look at the guide below to see the various levels.

ACTIVITY FACTOR

1.2 = sedentary (little or no exercise)

1.375 = light activity (light exercise/sports 1 to 3 days per week)

1.55 = moderate activity (moderate exercise/sports 4 to 5 days per week)

1.725 = very active (hard exercise/sports 6 to 7 days per week)

1.9 = extra active (very hard exercise/sports 6 to 7 days per week and physical job)

These activity factors have been known to overestimate true activity, so for this program I suggest you start off at the bottom with an activity factor of 1.2. If you're exercising above and beyond what's required for this program, your number might be 1.55 or higher. I would be surprised if anyone was at the extra active level. That's usually reserved for professional athletes or decathletes.

The final piece of the TDEE puzzle is multiplying your activity factor by your BMR.

Daily Maintenance Calories (TDEE) = BMR × Activity Factor

Your TDEE is your maintenance level when it comes to calorie intake. Let's say your TDEE is 2,000 calories a day. If you eat less than 2,000 calories a day, you're going to lose weight. Eat more than 2,000, and you'll gain weight. Calories in, calories out.

Now we can finally use the TDEE to figure out our daily calorie "budget," which is the key variable in the weight-loss formula. One pound of human fat is roughly equivalent to 3,500 calories. In order to lose one pound of fat each week, you'll need to be at a caloric deficit of 3,500 calories per week, which breaks down to 500 calories per day.

We'll stick with the 2,000 calorie daily budget from our TDEE example above. If you only eat 1,500 calories a day, then at the end of one week you should've lost a pound of fat based on our "calories in, calories out" principle. It could be slightly more or slightly less, but it should be close to one pound.

Congratulations—no more scary equations in this chapter!

ONE MISSTEP FORWARD, TWO BIG STEPS BACK

The problem is, is that you know, you think that he's helping you...but he's hurting you...

— SONNY BLACK

You've just learned nutrition's most important law—the Law of Energy Balance—and conquered the basics of counting calories. We'll adjust your daily calorie budget along the way as your weight drops and then again once you reach your goal, but for now, you're ready to roll.

Before we finish this chapter, I want to address a question I get asked a lot about calories in, calories out: If a deficit of 3,500 calories per week results in the loss of one pound of body fat, could someone go extremely low with their caloric intake and lose even more than that? Is it possible to lose ten pounds in two weeks if someone essentially doesn't eat?

Short answer: No.

Aside from the fact that weight loss is not linear, someone who tried this approach would find his body fighting against him. The human body is sophisticated; it knows if you're not eating enough, and it will try to hold on to that body fat for as long as possible. It's preserving that fat for another time when you might need it.

This is commonly referred to as "starvation mode." If you slash your calories too aggressively or go on a stupid diet where you're only drinking lemon cayenne water, your body is not going to let you cheat. Furthermore, you're not feeding your body the calories it needs for you to make it through rest days, let alone workout days.

My point is clear: don't try to be a hero. Fat loss is not linear, and it doesn't happen overnight. Slow and consistent fat loss is the only way you're going to have sustainable progress.

There's a chart in the macronutrient chapter (see chapter 5) that shows your estimated weight loss per week based on your body fat percentage, but I can tell you upfront that the maximum amount you can expect to lose when you're in a sensible caloric deficit is 1 to 1.5 pounds per week. If you're just starting out, you might lose more, and if you're super lean, you might lose less.

Either way, I can promise you that your body won't let you cheat the system. There are no shortcuts on the road to your ideal body, only hard work and patience.

Now that you know the ins and outs of calories in, calories out, let's tackle a subject that many of you might not be familiar with: intermittent fasting.

KEY TAKEAWAYS

○ Counting calories is a necessary evil that separates those who are truly lean from those who look skinny but are technically fat (skinny fat).

○ The Law of Energy Balance (Calories In vs. Calories Out) has the biggest impact on your nutrition.

○ People struggle with calories in two ways: underestimating the number of calories they eat and thinking they need more calories than they actually do.

○ Figuring out how many calories you burn every day comes from multiplying your basal metabolic rate by your daily activity factor.

○ A pound of body fat is roughly equivalent to 3,500 calories, so in order to lose a pound a week, you need to operate at a caloric deficit of 3,500 calories for the week.

○ If you slash your calories too aggressively, your body will go into starvation mode and do everything it can to hold on to that fat.

○ Sustainable fat loss is slow and steady.

○ Most people can expect to lose 1 to 1.5 pounds per week with *Hack Your Fitness*.

ACTION STEP

🏋 Calculate your basal metabolic rate (using the formula or Google), then multiply that by 1.2 (the appropriate daily activity factor for most people) to determine your daily maintenance calories.

CHAPTER 4

THE HUNGER GAMES: INTERMITTENT FASTING

As we grow older our biases and sense of superiority become an impediment or learning disability. We close off our minds to possibilities.

— ROBERT GREENE

Once again, I have to credit my wife for a pivotal moment in my fitness journey. I think she was both looking out for my success and fed up with cooking six meals a day when she stumbled upon intermittent fasting (IF) in 2011 courtesy of a friend's Facebook post.

"Honey, look at these pictures Ben posted," she said,

motioning me over to look at her computer. "He's trying intermittent fasting. Look at the results he got!"

The excitement in her voice was palpable over what she thought could be the missing puzzle piece for me. In fact, it was the missing piece, that final digit that needed to be rearranged in my sequence to fix the syntax error. I was just too brainwashed to see it after reading *Burn the Fat, Feed the Muscle* and committing to six meals a day.

"That's crazy!" I told her. "You can't not eat. Your metabolism will slow down and your body will go into starvation mode." Dejected, my wife clicked away from the photos and went back to browsing Facebook. Little did she know that my interest had been piqued. I was too proud to admit that my system wasn't working and hid my frustration often, but the reality was that I was desperate for one final change that would unlock the door for me.

I was tired of feeling hungry all the time and constantly thinking about my next meal. It's exhausting trying to work in double the number of meals a normal person eats, especially when you're tracking every calorie. I felt guilty that my wife was prepping so many meals only for me to be stuck on my double-digit body fat plateau.

A mixture of desperation and frustration pushed me toward intermittent fasting.

I started doing a ton of Web research on the subject, and it didn't take long for me to discover the two godfathers of intermittent fasting: Brad Pilon, who wrote *Eat Stop Eat*, and Martin Berkhan, who runs the website Leangains.com. We'll talk about them more in just a moment, but it was their work that inspired me to try IF for myself.

To say that something "totally changed my life" sounds dramatic. IF really did, though. My search for the perfect long-term diet was over. My syntax error was nearly solved.

So why did it take me so long to discover the truth?

PARADIGM SHIFT

We cannot solve problems by using the same kind of thinking when we created them.

— ALBERT EINSTEIN

Intermittent fasting has started to gain popularity in the past five to ten years. The *New York Times* actually ran a story on its website in March 2016 about Jimmy Kimmel crediting his weight-loss success to the 5:2 fasting protocol found in *Eat Stop Eat* (which we'll cover in detail later in the chapter).

For years, fasting carried a negative connotation in fitness circles. It wasn't until recently, when people started challenging everything in the nutrition world, that claims like "fasting deprives your body of nutrients" and "fasting isn't good for your health" were proven to be untrue. My friends, we're in the golden age of diet enlightenment.

As I explained in the introduction, the food and supplement industries share a common backdrop: advertising. Each of these industries rakes in billions annually by selling you not only their products but the belief that you can't get fit without them. The whole notion of fasting threatens the bottom line of these industries because they *want* you to eat.

Protein powders are marketed as a meal replacement because, when you're eating six meals a day like I was, some days you don't have time for one of your meals. Rather than skipping that meal, why not drink a protein shake to get the nutrients you need?

I spent years trapped in this cycle of marketing hype and misinformation. I stubbornly believed I held the golden ticket to body recomposition and kept running myself ragged with meal prep and ever-changing exercise programs. If I could just outwork my slow metabolism, I could achieve the body I wanted. All the while, I kept throwing money at food and supplement providers that were laughing all the way to the bank.

My wife's discovery of IF and my subsequent research pulled the wool off my eyes, and in that moment, I had to grapple with some truths I'd ignored for a long time:

- A fasted state shorter than twenty-four hours will not make your metabolism slow down.
- You don't have to eat six meals a day to get ripped.
- The food and supplement industries do not have your best interests at heart. They're only trying to promote and sell their products.

Here's the bottom line: being in a prolonged caloric restriction is the only proven nutritional method for consistent fat loss (Law of Energy Balance). And when you rule out liposuction, the most effective way to abide by this law and sustain that caloric restriction is with intermittent fasting. In my mind, this makes IF the most powerful dieting protocol that exists for people who share our goals.

It took me years to correct this part of my syntax error. I'm thrilled we get to dig into IF now and save you the frustration I felt prior to discovering this game changer.

IF 101

What got you here isn't going to get you there.

Let's start with a definition that's fundamental to understanding IF. What does it mean to fast? The definition I use is from *Eat Stop Eat*: "Fasting is the act of willingly abstaining from all food, and in some cases drink, for a predetermined period of time. The key word in this definition is 'willingly' as it is the difference between fasting and starving."

Before we continue, I want to clearly define one important thing. Intermittent fasting is not a diet. It has nothing to do with *what* you can eat; it has to do with *when* you can eat.

Intermittent fasting is a dieting *protocol* that splits your day into two windows: fasting and feeding. For IF to work, your fasting window has to be longer than your feeding window. That's a basic rule that you need to understand before you begin IF.

Nutritionally speaking, human beings are either in a fasted state or a fed state. It's like yin and yang. Your body is always in one state or the other, or transitioning between the two. When you eat food, it takes your body about eight

94 · HACK YOUR FITNESS

to ten hours to fully process that food. During that time following your last meal of the day, your body is in a fed state as that food is being processed. Once it's fully processed, your body enters a fasted state.

When you're in the fed state, your body gets all the nutrients it needs from the food you just ate and stores the excess calories it doesn't need. This means you're not going to burn any of your stored fat, since your body is sourcing energy directly from the food you just consumed. After eight to ten hours, your body has burned up all the energy that was in your bloodstream as you enter the fasted state. When you're in the fasted state, your body will search for energy to burn and will then turn to the calories that were stored to fat back when you were in the fed state.

There's a lot more science behind it, but very simply, if there's no food in your body, then the next source of energy that's available is the stored fat on your body. The end result here is that your body fat level will drop during the fasted state.

Now it should be clear why it is beneficial to work out during the fasted state. Rather than getting energy from food we've consumed, our body only has its stored fat supplies to burn.

But wait a minute. If our bodies are in a fed state for as long as eight to ten hours after we eat, why then do we feel hungry just three to four hours after eating? Remember those invisible scripts? Our bodies don't actually need the food; we're in a fed state and burning the energy from the food we just ate. If you can believe it, you feel hungry because your brain has been trained to feel hungry after three to four hours.

Our eating habits are so deeply ingrained in our minds that we don't think twice when our brain says to eat breakfast in the morning, get lunch around noon, and sit down for dinner in the evening. That's just the way society has been groomed. Eating habits are such a powerful force that we're not even aware of how it shapes our daily lives.

We're just like Pavlov's dogs. Every time the trainer rang the bell, the dogs would start salivating because they thought, "This is my trigger. I'm going to be fed soon." Human beings are exactly the same. We're conditioned to react when we see food, so when you see someone eating or smell delicious food, your pancreas will actually start producing insulin in anticipation of the meal that you're about to eat. Insulin is what breaks down the food, and when your body starts producing it, you feel hungry. Food is the human equivalent of Pavlov's bell.

The hormone that works in opposition to insulin is called glucagon. These two hormones work together to keep your glucose—or blood sugar—levels stable. When you eat, your blood sugar spikes, so the pancreas produces insulin to lower the level of glucose in your bloodstream. When you're in a fasted state and your blood sugar drops too low, glucagon is produced to raise the glucose level. Your body is very efficient that way.

We must understand insulin and glucagon production as it relates to insulin sensitivity. The more sensitive your body is to insulin, the more efficiently you will break down the foods that you eat, which means that less will be stored as fat. The opposite of insulin sensitivity is insulin resistance, which means your body does not produce as much insulin and more calories will be stored as body fat. Insulin resistance is the reason diabetics need to take an insulin shot before they eat. Their pancreas can't do the job by itself.

The key to fat loss is increasing your insulin sensitivity, thereby increasing how effective your body is at breaking down the calories. I bet you can guess the two times our insulin sensitivity is going to be the highest. Ding, ding, ding! You guessed it: insulin sensitivity is highest after a long fast and after a hard workout.

So, when you work out in the morning during a fasted

state, you're achieving the holy grail of fat burning. You're essentially taking a flamethrower to your stored body fat.

During the section on discipline in chapter 1, I advocated for having a treat after a heavy workout. When you're coming off a heavy workout, in a fasted state, with your insulin sensitivity at a high point, your body is going to burn food so efficiently that whatever you put in your mouth will go directly to muscle recovery. Very few of those calories will actually be stored as fat. Physiologically, it's the ideal time to have a treat.

Before we move on to the benefits and drawbacks of IF, I want to debunk this notion that if you don't eat, your body will start burning your muscles. There have been studies (which I've included in the reference section) that show that your body doesn't actually dig into your muscles until the third or fourth day of continued fasting. You're at no risk of losing your hard-earned muscles due to intermittent fasting. The only energy source getting burned during the fasting window is your stored body fat. You can rest assured that your muscles are safe.

LIFE IN THE FAST LANE: BENEFITS AND DRAWBACKS

It is difficult to get a man to understand something when his salary depends on his not understanding it.

— UPTON SINCLAIR

As the author of an honest fitness program, I like to show you all sides of the *Hack Your Fitness* system. This means looking at both the benefits and the drawbacks of IF. Let's start with the positives, which not surprisingly outweigh the negatives by a wide margin.

The first benefit you get from intermittent fasting is the immediate kicker, so to speak. The first week is rough because your body will be in shock and your brain will be ringing the dinner bell nonstop. Yet you're going to see results right out of the gate, which is a nice reward for your brain and helps solidify this new routine as a habit. You will immediately feel less bloated and full, and you may even look leaner right away.

The second benefit—and this was everything for me (and especially my wife)—is not having to worry about meal prep anymore. The mental and physical toll you endure when you're eating six meals a day is replaced with newfound free time and peace of mind. I'm only worried about eating two meals a day now, not six. That's why IF was such a game changer for me. For all the wives and girlfriends out there who handle meal prep—like mine used to do—IF is one of the best gifts your partner can give you. The days of silent resentment are over!

I also really enjoy the third benefit of intermittent fasting, which is getting to eat big. People who advocate six small meals a day claim that you never feel hungry because you end up eating all day. I'm just going to have to call bullshit on that notion right now. I was starving all day because I never felt full! After years of agony, I like to go big with my lunch and dinner now. I'm happy to say I walk away from the table full now and don't think about eating again until close to the next mealtime. The days of nonstop stomach rumbling are long gone.

If you're grinding out six meals a day right now, doesn't this life sound amazing?

At this point we need to pause and reiterate that IF is not some touted holy grail of fitness or a miracle diet, but merely a tool (albeit a powerful one) in your fitness repertoire to help you maintain a prolonged caloric restriction. The benefits from here on out get a bit theoretical, and many of them have not been proven by pure science, so take the next few in stride.

One of the claimed positive changes in your life resulting from IF has to do with changes to your growth hormone (GH), which helps your muscles grow. Studies show that there are times when your GH will spike, like after a good night's sleep or a strenuous workout. Your GH also spikes during your fasting windows.

GH isn't just for growing muscles; it also counteracts cortisol, the stress hormone. When you're stressed out, your body releases cortisol and begins storing more fat. By countering the effects of cortisol, GH is basically helping you store less body fat.

Intermittent fasting has also been shown to reduce inflammation, which is linked to a whole slew of health problems. Your appetite will also decrease during IF thanks to the stabilization of an enzyme called ghrelin that's found in your stomach lining and stimulates your appetite. By stabilizing ghrelin, IF minimizes that feeling of being hungry.

On the far end of the spectrum, there are a handful of studies that claim that intermittent fasting can even help cure cancer. I would definitely take that one with a grain of salt.

For me, avoiding the meal prep and being able to eat big are the two biggest advantages of IF, and they gave me enough of a reason to give IF a shot. Eating big was a huge key to the sustainability of this program for me. Our bodies crave that feeling of being full so much that any system that allows us to feel that way has a good chance of sticking around.

I've been doing intermittent fasting for six years now. This is my life. There's no "getting off" this diet for me. I can never go back to eating and living how I was before IF. The benefits are too great, and the rewards are definitely worth the sacrifice.

Now, that all said, there are some drawbacks to intermittent fasting. One of the sticking points is that studies have been inconclusive regarding the effects of IF on women, whose bodies react differently than men when their hormones, insulin, and glucagon levels change. Plenty of women have found success with IF, and others have been unsuccessful.

My advice to women is to give intermittent fasting a try and see for yourself. There are two obvious disclaimers here: consult a physician if you have any physical ailments or diabetes, and don't attempt IF if you're pregnant. If you're a healthy woman who's not expecting, it's not going to hurt to try it. If it works for you, stick with it, and if it doesn't, you can stop. Whether the results are good or bad, please let me know about your experience!

Regardless of gender, the second big drawback is that

your first week of intermittent fasting is going to suck. I'm not going to sugarcoat it for you. Your body will be in a state of shock because it's accustomed to three square meals a day at specific times; the long fasting window will set off alarm bells in your brain telling you that you're starving and you have to eat. If you need something in the morning, I'd suggest drinking black coffee, which has zero calories, or chewing a piece sugar-free gum (little to no calories).

The final drawback is actually a myth we're going to debunk. If you're worried that your blood sugar will drop due to IF and you'll pass out, research says not to worry. I included two studies in the reference section of this book that explain how your blood sugar levels don't drop until ten to twelve hours after you've eaten, which is the whole fasting window. So right around the time you would need to worry about a drop, it's time for lunch.

As daunting as IF seems during that first week, I would encourage you by saying that the human body is very adaptable. The same way that Pavlov trained his dogs, you can train your body with your mind to curb hunger during certain times of the day.

Soon the weeks will turn into months, and intermittent fasting will be part of your routine. In order to decide what

IF will look like for you, let's examine four of the most popular protocols.

ALL FASTS LEAD TO ROME

Making lots of tiny choices depletes one's subsequent self-control.

— DR. KATHLEEN VOHS

I consider Brad Pilon to be one of the godfathers of the IF movement since his book *Eat Stop Eat* really got the ball rolling and helped IF gain awareness on a larger scale. I would highly encourage you to read Brad's book. It's a mere seventy pages long and packed with myths of the fitness industry that Brad debunks. It really opened my eyes the first time I read it.

That said, I actually don't follow Brad's protocol, which is called "5:2." It was too difficult for me to adopt on a consistent basis. His approach requires you to do one or two full twenty-four-hour fasts every week, and the rest of the time you eat normally. That's why it's eat, stop, eat.

However, these aren't twenty-four-hour periods where you skip breakfast, lunch, and dinner. Brad recognizes that psychologically it's easier to skip breakfast than it is dinner, so his method calls for a big dinner the night before your fast, then not eating until the next day's dinner. By shifting your hours around, you're only skipping breakfast and lunch.

I prefer Martin Berkhan's system, which he outlines at Leangains.com, because it's more geared toward people who want to fast and work out. In fitness parlance, Martin's protocol is referred to as "16:8" as it includes a sixteen-hour fast and an eight-hour feeding window.

The easiest way I can think to manage a sixteen-hour fast is by skipping breakfast. My last meal at night is dinner, which I finish around 8:00 p.m. I won't eat again until lunch the next day at noon. That's sixteen hours. During my feeding window from noon to 8:00 p.m., I'll have a big lunch and a big dinner so I'm satiated all the way until lunch the next day.

I recommend checking out Martin's website if you want to learn more about IF. He's a nutritional consultant and a fitness guru, so his website is chock-full of great information. Like I mentioned earlier, his website and Brad's book were my two go-to resources when I started researching IF and was still very skeptical about whether I should try it.

The third protocol that's gained some popularity comes from Ori Hofmekler's book *The Warrior Diet*. In IF parlance, the Warrior Diet is known as "20/4" since it's a twenty-hour fast followed by a four-hour feeding window.

It might seem counterintuitive to eat as the ancient warriors once did, but the reasoning behind this protocol makes a lot of sense. You see, warriors spent their whole day out at battle only to return to camp at night for dinner, their one large meal of the day.

You don't see too many overweight warriors, now do you?

The last popular IF protocol I want to mention is alternate day fasting (ADF). This is similar to Brad's protocol but involves fasting every other day. In other words, you eat for twenty-four hours, and you fast for twenty-four hours. How you structure your fasting window is up to you.

Personal preference will dictate which protocol you choose, but for me, I only like to use a twenty-four-hour fast when I know I have a big event like Thanksgiving coming up. I pride myself on having good mental discipline, but to go for twenty-four hours without food multiple times a week is too challenging even for me. In those rare instances when I do fast for twenty-four hours, I find that those last four hours from 4:00 to 8:00 p.m. drag on for an eternity.

I can't advocate a program that makes me want to eat my

own arm four hours a day, three to four days a week. That's not a recipe for long-term success with IF.

For happy fitness, I recommend Martin's 16:8 protocol. You consume no calories for sixteen hours, eat a big lunch and dinner, and then don't eat again until lunch. It's straightforward and sustainable. As long as you stay under ten calories during your fasting window, you won't derail. Sugar-free gum, black coffee (with a splash of milk if needed), and sparkling water will become your go-to hunger hacks as you adjust during that difficult first week.

The key I've found to surviving your fasting window is to stay busy. I'm an early riser, so I wake up around 4:00 a.m. every day and do about an hour and a half of work in the morning. I then work out from 6:00 a.m. to 7:00 a.m., shower up, and head into the office. I'm at my desk by 7:30 a.m. and focused on cranking out my deliverables while other people are still out getting breakfast. Food is the last thing I'm thinking about when I'm busting my ass at the office.

After remaining disciplined throughout the morning, your feeding window represents a glorious part of your day. There is a lot of flexibility as to how you spend your calories during that eight-hour stretch. If you're a foodie, you can look forward to any meal that fits your calorie budget and hits the necessary macros. You know how to count calories now. Once we cover macro tracking, I'm going to turn you loose and let you find your own way in this brave new world of diet and nutrition. You'll develop a custom system that works just for you as you progress in your journey.

Let's say you have 1,500 calories to "spend" during your feeding window. It doesn't matter how you spend them as long as you don't go over 1,500. Like I said earlier, I prefer a big lunch because I'm coming off a fast and I'm hungry. Then I follow that up with a big dinner.

Other people like to spread the calories out and snack throughout their feeding window. I still recommend two or three big meals just because it's hard to keep track of what you're eating when you're snacking for eight hours. It's so mindless that what starts out as a few chips keeps going until you've eaten the whole bag without realizing it. Eating two or three meals during your feeding window is easier all around.

If I had to use one word to describe my experience with IF since 2011, it would be "freedom." I'm free of time-consuming meal prep, free of guilt for asking my wife to undertake said meal prep, free of never feeling full, free of the anger I felt for years over why I could never sustain single-digit body fat, and free of the marketing machine's lies.

I was a skeptic at first, but after researching, reading Brad's book, and personally testing IF, I can say without hesitation that it's been a life-changing experience. My whole thought process regarding fitness and nutrition changed when I allowed myself to break away from the notions I'd clung to for years. It was a paradigm shift, a true moment of personal growth.

I have IF to thank for so many milestones in my fitness journey, but most importantly, it single-handedly improved my relationship with my wife because she no longer has to spend half the day prepping my meals. Seeing as how she's motivated the majority of my major turning points with fitness, I at least owe her that much.

The one final question you may be asking is, "Do I absolutely *have* to do intermittent fasting in order to hack fitness?" If you've learned anything in the last two chapters, you will know that the answer is no. You don't have to do IF to get results. I'm simply staying true to my original promise, and that is to provide you with the simplest, straightest line to success based on my years of struggle, research, and experiences helping hundreds of people along the way. If you can't stand the thought of skipping breakfast and are fine with eating three smaller meals over the course of the day, rest assured that as long as you abide by the Law of Energy Balance, you will still be able to find success at the end of this road.

That's it for intermittent fasting. The next step in your education is learning the second Law of Nutrition, which is the Law of Macronutrient Balance. Fair warning: There will be some math.

KEY TAKEAWAYS

○ Fasting had been brushed aside as unhealthy for years by the food and supplement industries because not eating threatens their bottom lines.

○ Fasting for twenty-four hours or less will not slow down your metabolism.

○ You don't have to eat six meals a day to get fit.

○ Intermittent fasting (IF) is the most effective way to maintain a caloric deficit over a long period of time.

○ Fasting is willingly abstaining from food and/or drink for a predetermined period of time.

○ IF is not a diet that dictates what you can eat, but rather a schedule for when you can eat.

○ Your day is split into two windows with IF—fasting and feeding—with the fasting window being longer than the feeding window.

○ Your body is in a fed state for eight to ten hours after you eat. Once the food energy is processed, your body enters a fasted state.

○ You only burn food energy during a fed state. During a fasted state, your body sources energy from stored fat.

○ We get hungry even when our bodies are in a fed state because of our deeply ingrained, invisible eating scripts that dictate much of our behavior.

- A long fast and a hard workout increases your insulin sensitivity, which makes your body more effective at breaking down calories.
- Your body burns stored body fat in a fasted state, not your muscles.
- Some benefits of IF are that you see immediate results and your days of endless meal prep are over. Also, when you eat, you get to eat big.
- The drawbacks of IF are that results with women have been inconclusive and the first week really sucks.
- Right around the time you'd need to worry about a blood sugar drop with IF, it's time for your next meal.
- There are four IF protocols, and for the purposes of this program, I recommend 16:8.
- With 16:8, eating two or three meals during your feeding window is recommended compared to snacking because big meals are easier to track.
- You don't have to use IF to see results with *Hack Your Fitness* as long as you abide by the Laws of Nutrition, particularly the Law of Energy Balance.

ACTION STEPS

- Decide which IF protocol is best for you, and begin practicing it.
- To make things easier, decide before you start IF which hunger hacks you're going to employ and how you'll keep yourself busy during the times when you'd usually be eating.

CHAPTER 5

CHANGES AT THE MARGIN: MACRONUTRIENT MANIPULATION

Big doors swing on little hinges.

— W. CLEMENT STONE

"Changes at the margin" is a financial term for the tiny changes a company makes in their business that increase their margins significantly. It's another way of saying that the smallest changes you make can have a big impact. For me, macronutrient tracking was one of those tiny changes that greatly impacted my margins. It was the final number in my diet and nutrition syntax that needed reordering.

Even after counting calories and discovering intermittent fasting, this was the variable in the equation that got me from low-teens body fat to single digits and enabled me to maintain single digits. I consider it an essential cog in the *Hack Your Fitness* machine.

So just what the hell are macros? Here's the definition from the McKinley Health Center in Illinois: "Macronutrients are nutrients that provide calories or energy. Nutrients are substances needed for growth, metabolism, and other bodily functions. Since 'macro' means large, macronutrients are nutrients needed in large amounts."

Micronutrients are defined by the CDC as "nutrients that our body needs in smaller amounts, and that includes vitamins and minerals. Micronutrients are not produced in the body and must be derived from the diet." Basically, micronutrients are your vitamins, and macronutrients are energy that comes from anything that you eat.

Now that you've learned about counting calories and calculated your daily calorie budget or TDEE, you know how much you should be eating on a daily basis. In the scope of your diet and nutrition, that's the broad strokes. Macronutrients look at the specific foods you eat on a more granular level.

It's time to learn the second Law of Nutrition, which is the

Law of Macronutrient Balance. It states that finding the correct balance of macronutrients (protein, carbohydrates, and fat) is the key to rapid body recomposition.

Every calorie that enters your body through food is composed of a combination of the three macronutrients: protein, carbohydrates, and fat. Let's run through why each one is important.

Other than water, protein is the most abundant nutrient in the body. Protein has a whole host of functions within the body. It replaces old cells; helps build muscles, organs, blood, nails, hair, skin, and tissues; and assists in the formation of hormone antibodies and enzymes. Without proper protein intake, your body will slowly begin to shut down.

Carbohydrates are the body's preferred source of energy. Carbs are broken down to smaller versions called glucose, which we talked about in the previous chapter. All cells in the human body depend on glucose, as do the brain and nervous system for proper functioning.

Fat gets a bad rap, but it accomplishes many things. It gives us energy and provides protection within our body because it surrounds the vital organs. It takes part in cellular function and structure, regulates hormonal production, and balances body temperature.

Some foods fall at one extreme of macronutrient composition or the other.

Think about 100 grams of skinless chicken breast. You're looking at 23 grams of protein, zero carbs, and 1.24 grams of fat. Because it's a lean protein, there's very little fat.

At the other extreme you have 100 grams of white rice, for instance. Rice is almost all carbs with little to no fat and a small amount of protein. The macronutrient breakdown is 28 grams of carbs, less than 1 gram of fat, and 2.66 grams of protein. These numbers match pretty well with our perception of rice as a starchy carb.

There's a very simple formula for calculating calories if you know the macronutrient composition of a certain food. All you have to do is remember 4-4-9. For one gram of protein, there are four calories. For one gram of carbs, there are also four calories. For one gram of fat, there are nine calories. The important takeaway from this formula is that one gram of fat has more than double the calories in either protein or carbs. It's much denser calorically.

The FDA requires all foods to have a nutrition label on the back that gives the calorie count and the breakdown of macronutrients. Now that you know this formula, you can actually pick up any food and test it out. Using 4-4-9, you should come very close to the calorie number at the top. Pay attention to the servings, because when you look at the label, sometimes the amount of calories is per serving and not per package. There might be twelve servings in one package, but they'll only break it down per serving (another sly trick that many food companies use to prey on innocent consumers).

Macronutrients might seem too technical or too "mathy" for some people. Personally I was turned off by this portion of the diet at first. For many years I told myself I wasn't going to track food down to that level. It felt like overkill and seemed hard to stick with consistently.

But my stubbornness in this area prevented me from achieving the shredded state I always wanted. Once I actually took the plunge, I realized I was fretting over nothing substantial. The math behind tracking macros is so easy a first grader could do it. Once you know the 4-4-9 formula, that battle is half over. The next step is finding the correct ratio, or balance, of macronutrients in order to unlock *rapid body recomposition*.

YOUR BODY NEEDS BALANCE: WHY FAD DIETS FAIL

*I don't throw darts at a board. I bet on sure things. Read
Sun-Tzu, The Art of War. Every battle is won before it is
ever fought.*

— GORDON GEKKO

The human body always knows exactly what it needs.

If the goal is to lose body fat and get shredded, there's an
ideal amount of protein, carbs, and fat that your body will
need to reach that point. It's quite literally a formula. Every
person's formula will be slightly different, but luckily for
you, *Hack Your Fitness* includes a starting level where
everyone will see success right out of the gate. Later on,
we'll tweak this starting level and track things to make
sure everyone's formula is correct for him or her.

Fad diets like Atkins and the South Beach Diet appear at
first glance to follow a winning formula. All those before-
and-after photos show people enjoying immediate success.
If you've ever been on one of these diets, you know they
include a caloric restriction that will eventually lead to
weight loss courtesy of the "calories in, calories out" formula.

The question then is this: Why do these diets work temporarily but not long-term?

As you might expect, the problem has to do with the formulas used by these fad diets. Because these diets restrict the types of food you can eat, your body is not getting the necessary protein, carbs, and fat it needs for sustainable body recomposition. In contrast, the *Hack Your Fitness* diet does in fact restrict your calorie intake overall, but as far as food choices go, there's a lot more freedom.

Now would be a good time to explain the final Law of Nutrition, which is the Law of Food Choices. It states that for the purposes of body recomposition, the nutritional value of food makes little difference. Yes, really...but it's not as simple as you think. Let me explain why.

Intermittent fasting restricts the time you can eat, and macro tracking demands that your meals be comprised of certain types of foods, but within that framework, you can eat whatever the hell you want. I'm not going to say you can't eat this or you can only eat that. Armed with the knowledge of "garbage in, garbage out," you should feel empowered to make good food choices. I've included a *Hack Your Diet* guide with "good" and "bad" foods in the appendix, but for now, just keep in mind 4-4-9 and you'll be in good shape.

One of the earlier sections in this book was titled "Smoke and Mirrors." As you start down this road with *Hack Your*

Fitness, you're going to see some attractive lies that tempt you to jump ship and take the easier road promised by programs that claim your six-pack can come with a steady supply of burgers and fries. Don't believe this bullshit for one second.

These claims are either outright lies or half-truths. Can you start out this program eating junk food once a week and not fall off the wagon? Possibly. Can the *foundation* of your diet include burgers, fries, pizza, and milkshakes? Absolutely not. It's impossible to achieve long-term success with these kinds of foods as part of your diet.

But I thought you said calories in, calories out?

Here is the problem: when you eat fatty junk food, the caloric density is so high that one slice of pizza is going to be the equivalent of half of a pound of lean chicken breast, plus a baked potato and a whole plate of vegetables. When you're working out hard on a caloric deficit, you want to feel satiated after your meal and not crave a snack two hours later. If you have a choice to eat one slice of pizza or a full, wholesome meal that's going to fill you up, you're always going to opt for what makes you full. Nobody gets full off of one slice of pizza.

Back in chapter 3 we suggested that a good way to visualize

your calories for the day is to picture it as a budget. Every day, you have to choose how you spend your calories. Sure, you can eat a burger on a rest day—when your caloric intake is reduced—and still be within your budget. But that's it. With the number of calories in that burger, you're done for the day. No matter how hungry you get, you can't eat anything else.

Wouldn't it be smarter to choose two large plates of broccoli and "spend" only 100 calories? You'll be decently full afterward and still have plenty of calories left in your daily budget. I'm a sucker for junk food just like anyone else, but the calories just aren't worth the temporary satisfaction I get from indulgence. I'd rather feel full than satisfy my short-term cravings.

Without a doubt, the comment I hear the most from people after I teach them about proper nutrition and replacing the junk in their diet with wholesome foods is how full they feel all the time.

"I can't believe how much food I have to eat on the *Hack Your Fitness* program. Are you sure this is right?"

Yes, I'm sure. While it may seem like much more food than you are used to eating, calorically you are actually eating much less. Natural foods are lean and less dense than the junk you are used to gorging on.

So when you see a fad diet promising sustained success, or come across an ad for the "pizza and burgers" weight-loss program, just remember that there are no shortcuts between here and single-digit body fat. You have to pay the toll to drive on that road.

MACROS IN ACTION

Luck is what happens when preparation meets opportunity.

– SENECA

Now it's time to set up your macronutrient guidelines. Since tracking macros is tedious, we're going to front-load the work. Once we figure out what your macros are, I suggest you find a few easy and convenient meals that are within your parameters and that you love eating. Maybe love is a bit of an overstatement—find meals that you don't mind eating. Once you log this handful of meals in and track them, you can keep going back to them to lather, rinse, and repeat. They're your fallback or go-to options, or "Hacker Friendly" meals as I like to call them.

I have a place in Hong Kong where I eat lunch two or three times a week. Whenever I go, I always get the "Healthy Chicken Breast Meal" because I know the exact calories and the macros. I've already crunched the numbers, so I don't even have to think about what I'm eating. I can just enjoy my meal.

We're getting ahead of ourselves, though. Let's start our macronutrient manipulation by reviewing what we know. We calculated our total daily energy expenditure (TDEE). We remember that one pound of fat is 3,500 calories, which means that if we want to lose one pound of fat per week, we need to be at a caloric deficit of 3,500 calories per week.

We also know that we're going to be working out three days a week and resting four days. Our macros and calories will be manipulated in such a way that we're going to eat more calories on workout days, and on rest days, we're going to eat less. This strategy makes sense from both a psychological and a physiological standpoint.

After you work out, your body needs more energy to replenish and repair your muscles. On rest days, your body doesn't need as much energy, because you're not as active. Being able to eat more on a workout day is also a nice psychological reward.

I'll use myself as an example to explain how it works. If I were on a *Hack Your Fitness* prescribed cut, my maintenance level for workout days (three times a week) would be 2,000 calories a day. On rest days (four times a week), I consume roughly 60 percent of my maintenance calories, or 1,125 calories per day. Add everything up, and I'm at a weekly deficit of around 3,500 calories, or one pound of fat. (What can I say? I love my six-pack!)

So what about for you? Here's what you need to do. Remember the TDEE you calculated back at the end of chapter 3? Take that number and multiply it by seven. This will give you your *weekly* maintenance calorie level.

Now, as we know, one pound of fat equals 3,500 calories, so take that *weekly* number and subtract 3,500. This is your new calorie budget for the week, since you want to be losing roughly one pound of fat per week. Finally, you need to add in calorie cycling to the mix. On your three training days, you will be eating at the maintenance level, or your TDEE. On your four rest days, your calories will be slashed so you can hit that deficit of 3,500 calories per week. Use this formula to figure out your rest day calories:

Rest Day Calories = [Total Weekly Calories - (3 × TDEE)] / 4

With all these data points in our back pocket, we're ready to tackle macros. On both workout and rest days, protein will constitute 45- to 55 percent of your calories. I'll explain why it's kept so high in just a bit. On workout days, your protein is 45 percent, carbs 40 percent, and fat 15 percent of total calories consumed. You're going high carbs, low fat on workout days. On rest days, protein will be 55 percent, carbs 20 percent, and fat 25 percent.

I've found that for people who are new to this program and trying to learn everything, this is the easiest place to start with macros. You're probably going to tweak it at some point as you begin tracking and seeing results. Each person is a little bit different, and it is important to iterate our Minimum Effective Fitness Protocol often to ensure results.

Using myself again as an example, we can use 4-4-9 to see my breakdown for workout days: 225 grams of protein, 200 grams of carbs, and 33 grams of fat, for a total of 2,000 calories. On rest days, it's 155 grams of protein, 56 grams of carbs, and 30 grams of fat, for 1,150 calories. There's quite a big difference between workout days and rest days.

When people talk about calorie cycling, this is essentially what they mean. We're cycling the amount of calories we eat based on when we work out. On workout days, we eat more calories in the form of carbs than on rest days because our bodies needs more energy to recover.

The appropriate daily protein intake is actually a controversial issue within the nutrition field. I've included studies in the reference section that show why high protein intake levels are not bad for you. As a general rule, experts say the amount of protein you eat should be around 1.25 grams per pound of body weight.

Researchers acknowledge that protein is more important when you're in a caloric deficit because it has the effect of keeping you more satiated after meals. Because of its composition, protein takes a long time for your body to process. When you eat a loaf of bread versus a slab of meat, you'll feel hungry sooner because it takes less time for your body to process the bread than it does the hunk of protein.

When eating protein, you'll always want to include some sort of complex carbohydrate. Starchy carbs such as a baked potato or brown rice work great, as do veggies. We do this because our body breaks down protein the best (slowest) with carbohydrates. These complex carbs serve as a time-release function and feed our muscles the protein over a longer period of time, which is what we want.

One word of caution I want to throw out here is that macros are a bit counterintuitive. When you tell someone who is eating "healthy" but who doesn't know a thing about macros that you're eating carbs, fat, and protein every day, it's natural for that person to tell you, "Carbs are bad. You need to eat salads every day for every meal, and fat's bad, so you shouldn't eat fat, either." I should know because I was guilty of this for years. I forced myself to eat salads all the time and assumed it had to be healthier than meat.

This is where I remind you that your body needs everything.

The secret sauce is in finding the right combination of the three macronutrients so that your body can operate at optimal efficiency. Fat is not bad for you if you eat the right amount. Of course, there are good fats like olive oil and bad fats like the oil used to fry French fries. The same goes for good carbs and bad carbs. (If you're curious about good and bad food choices, check out the *Hack Your Diet* guide in the appendix.)

Another word of caution: Fat creeps up really fast. At more than double the caloric density of the other two macronutrients (4-4-9), fat deserves extra attention in your budget. Spend fat wisely.

Whew! Is your head spinning yet? I want you to take a few minutes right now and calculate your macros for your training days and rest days. It's a lot of math, but trust me, this is the most critical step to solving the nutrition puzzle and an absolute requirement for unveiling those abs you've always wanted to show off.

I know what you're thinking: "This is too much math!" Don't worry. We've got you covered. The whole point of this program is to simplify and streamline your fitness, which is why I've created a free macro calculator for you to download as a special bonus for taking this final step seriously.

Go to http://hackyour.fitness/resources and download the Macro Calculator. All you have to do is punch in your age, weight, and height in centimeters, and the calculator will spit out the exact training day and rest day calculations for you. How's that for efficiency?

THE ONLY WAY IS TO WEIGH

The most valuable commodity I know of is information.

— GORDON GEKKO

As I mentioned, tracking macros is very tedious at the beginning. But if you're willing to get down to this level of detail, then I guarantee you will be successful.

We're going to make things easy by front-loading the work and finding a few meals during this period that are your go-to "Hacker Friendly" meals. You need these fallback options because it's just not sustainable to sit down and weigh your food, track your macros, and crunch the numbers at every single meal for the rest of your life. Eventually you're going to be too lazy to do that, or you'll feel self-conscious about it when someone makes a comment during a family dinner as you bust out your food scale. You do it once or twice, find your foods, log your numbers, and then, boom, you can go to them consistently.

For tracking everything, the best mobile app out there is MyFitnessPal by Under Armour. (See appendix for a detailed, step-by-step setup guide). I've tested it out and can vouch for it, but I'm more of an old-school guy and use a manual spreadsheet to track my macros (I blame my finance background). I have many friends and coaching clients who use MyFitnessPal and swear by it. The key is to find a tracking method that you can stick with.

In order to track your macros, you need a food scale. I use a Joseph Joseph scale that is compact and good for travel, but there are many cheaper options. It doesn't matter the brand or the price; you just need a food scale that works.

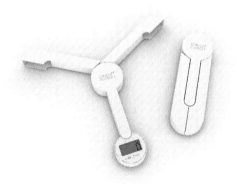

Joseph Joseph TriScale™ (www.josephjoseph.com)

I recommend bringing a lot of different foods home and weighing them so you develop a sense of the macronutrient composition and caloric density in various foods that you might eat.

Let's say you have a chicken breast you got from the store that weighs 100 grams. Your next step is to jump online and Google search "calories in 100 grams of chicken breast." Two websites you'll see among the results are CalorieKing.com and FatSecret.com. Either is fine. From Fat Secret, you'll find that 100 grams of chicken breast has 23 grams of protein, zero carbs, and 1.24 grams of fat, for 110 calories.

Let's double-check that using the 4-4-9 method: 23 grams of protein × 4 = 92 calories, and 1.24 grams of fat × 9 = 11.16 calories. Add those together, and you get 103.16, which is close to the calories listed. Again, this formula gives us approximate caloric values, so a difference of 6.84 calories is acceptable.

Every website has a different calculation for chicken breast. The key is to pick one website and stick with it for all your foods. Your numbers will be off if you switch back and forth.

Tracking macros is no more complex than weighing and researching various foods. Make it easy on yourself by taking a day before you start this program and weighing every item on the *Hack Your Diet* food list that you might potentially eat. Log those numbers in your app or spreadsheet, and then all you'll need for tracking is the food weight. By building up a massive database ahead of time, you'll increase your knowledge and decrease the number of times you need to use the food scale. Eventually you'll be able to eyeball a piece of meat or a plate of veggies and know roughly how many grams you've got.

Anyone can go to the gym and work out, calculate how many calories they're eating, or even do intermittent fasting. But it is getting down to this very detailed level of calculating the exact combination of macronutrients that you're putting into your body that separates the elite from the average. This is the true *Hack Your Fitness* litmus test.

DUMP SUPPLEMENTS, AND CHEW YOUR CALORIES

How long are you going to wait before you demand the best for yourself...?

— EPICTETUS

I've already detailed the true intentions of the supplement industry, but from a nutritional standpoint, a lot of the supplements you get off the shelf just don't deliver the benefits they advertise. I speak from years of firsthand experience and frustration.

You don't just have to take my word for it, though. Mike Matthews runs the popular fitness websites MuscleFor-Life.com and LegionAthletics.com, and he agreed to act as a resource for *Hack Your Fitness*. Mike extensively tested various supplements in the lab, and the results were eye-popping. Here are some takeaways from the article he wrote for his website, titled "The Absolute Best (and Worst) Supplements for Muscle Growth":

- Most supplements that claim to aid in muscle growth do absolutely nothing.
- The vast majority of testosterone boosters are completely worthless because they rely on ineffective ingredients and/or produce negligible testosterone increases.
- Finally, I'll directly quote my personal favorite: "Protein powder doesn't directly help you build muscle faster. Eating enough protein does."

I find supplements unnecessary, so I don't use them. Furthermore, I always advocate chewing your calories when you're in a caloric deficit so you feel full for longer. The only times I recommend drinking a protein shake is on your workout days when you're feeling super full but need to get your last bit of protein in for the day. In that case, have a protein shake so you can hit your numbers.

If you do decide to use protein shakes, make sure to get

them from Mike. After seeing the shoddy quality of the products he tested, Mike was inspired to create his own supplement line called LEGION. His stuff is the real deal. His website LegionAthletics.com is also a great resource for any kind of fitness research.

Along the same lines, I'd recommend a simple multivitamin to help with micronutrients, and that's it. You don't need whatever else is being sold out of your local Vitamin Shoppe or GNC.

MY TYPICAL MEALS

You have to assemble your life yourself—action by action.

— MARCUS AURELIUS

As an example, below are two of my typical days on this program. Notice my strict adherence to the macro ratios of 45 percent protein, 40 percent carbs, and 15 percent fat on workout days, and 55 percent protein, 20 percent carbs, and 25 percent fat on rest days. I also have flexibility and variety with my meal plans. My calorie intake and macros are 99 percent on point, and I'm still allowed to have rice, bread, potatoes, sashimi, and even cookies. You don't have to eat dried chicken every day.

Workout Day - Meal 1	Quantity	Calories	Protein	Carbs	Fat
Healthy Chicken Breast (skinless)	200g	280	46	0	2
Bell Peppers	60g	12	0.54	2.76	0.06
Brown Rice	85g	108	2.5	22.5	1
Black Beans	30g	102	6.3	18.9	0.27
Quest Protein Chips	32g	120	21	5	2
Lenny & Larry's Complete Cookie	1 cookie	360	16	50	12
Totals		982	92.34	99.16	17.33

Workout Day - Meal 2	Quantity	Calories	Protein	Carbs	Fat
Egg Whites	24	412	86	5.75	1.34
Broccoli	100g	30	2.4	5.8	0.4
Sweet Potato	162g	139	2.6	32.4	0.2
Vanilla Protein Powder	1.5 scoop	180	34.5	4.5	3
Low fat soy milk	12 oz.	90	6	9	3
Quest Bar	1 bar	200	20	21	9
Totals		1051	151.5	78.45	16.94

Grand Total		2033	244	178	34

Rest Day - Meal 1	Quantity	Calories	Protein	Carbs	Fat
Low Fat Cottage Cheese	452g	400	56	16	10
Bell Peppers	60g	12	0.54	2.76	0.06
Quest Protein Chips	32g	120	21	5	2
Totals		532	77.54	23.76	12.06

Rest Day - Meal 2	Quantity	Calories	Protein	Carbs	Fat
Salmon Sashimi	10 pieces	410	61.3	0	16.8
1 Small Baked Potato	138g	129	3.5	29	0.2
Mango	195g	120	1.6	20	0.8
Totals		659	66.4	49	17.8

Grand Total		1191	144	73	30

Tracking macros can actually be fun, believe it or not. Think of it as a daily puzzle that you have to solve—a treasure hunt to find the right combinations of foods to hit your numbers every day. Each element of each meal is another piece to the puzzle. The satisfaction you get when nailing your macros spot on at the end of the day is a simple but meaningful reward. You probably think I'm crazy, but I guarantee you will feel the same once you try it for yourself!

Look at this sample menu, consult the *Hack Your Diet* guide in the appendix, and find the right balance for you. That's the only way you will be able to sustain this diet long-term.

You have to enjoy what you eat. Even though you're not having a burger, these meals can include tasty foods that you feel you can eat over and over again. This is the key to sustainability. These meals are going to be the building blocks of your diet for the duration of your program.

WHAT FAT LOSS LOOKS LIKE

Only the educated are free.

— EPICTETUS

Here's the million-dollar question you've been waiting to ask: "How much fat will I lose, and how quickly will I lose it?"

It's the reason we're all here—single-digit body fat and that elusive six-pack. Depending on your starting body fat percentage, your initial results will vary. Take a look at the chart below to see what your results might look like:

Bodyfat %	Expected Loss
> 20%	-2.0 lbs/week
18-19%	-1.7 lbs/week
15-17%	-1.5 lbs/week
12-14%	-1.3 lbs/week
9-11%	-1.0 lbs/week
<8%	-0.7 lbs/week

As you lose fat, there are a couple of things to keep in mind. First, fat loss is not linear. Don't miss this one! These are just guidelines. If you're losing a pound a week, it's not going to be consistently a pound a week, every single week. Fat loss zig-zags on the way down. Even if you're 100 percent compliant with your diet and you're doing your lifts, your fat loss is not going to be linear, because that's just the way the human body operates. After three or four weeks of consistent fat loss, many people will hit a plateau.

I experienced a plateau firsthand during my first cut, back in 2008. I had read Venuto's book, and I was working out like crazy. At the outset I was losing a pound and a half every week consistently, then from weeks four to six, my fat loss stalled. I plateaued.

I panicked and made a mistake in how I responded. I was doing an hour of lifting and an hour of cardio every day. I decided to double down on my cardio, which is actually the wrong thing to do tactically in the long run. I came dangerously close to burning myself out. This is a common mistake a lot of people make when facing a dreaded plateau. They overreact, end up overworking their bodies, and burn themselves out.

Fortunately for me, in the middle of week six, my weight actually plunged almost four pounds. My body made up the ground it lost during those two weeks when I stalled. That's how these things work. You're going to start off hot and then hit stretches where you're not losing.

Why is this the case? At any given moment there are a number of factors that affect your fat-burning progress, with the most relevant one being water retention. On an aggressive fat-burning program, your body is actively breaking down the triglycerides that are held up in your fat cells for energy. As you burn these off, certain fat cells do not always shrink immediately but are temporarily filled with water. What that means is that sometimes even after you've burned off those fat cells, they won't shrink until much later, which results in a plateau in body weight. You need to trust the system, exercise patience, and have faith in science. Your weekly fat loss will fluctuate over time, but on average, if you stick with it, you're going to lose between a pound and a pound and a half until you hit single-digit body fat.

On the technical side, you should use the same scale and weigh in at the same time every day. I suggest weighing in first thing in the morning when you haven't eaten in hours and your hydration level hasn't changed as it does throughout your day. Whatever time you choose, be consistent. Consistency is a tenant of *Hack Your Fitness*.

For measuring body fat, there are several methods available, but for our purposes of convenience and cost (we're hackers after all), the body fat calipers remain the most economical and accurate method that is widely available. I recommend Accu-Measure Fitness body fat calipers, which cost under twenty dollars and can be used in the convenience of your own home.

The most accurate measurement is the hydrostatic weighing method, but it's an involved process and quite costly. You're weighed on land, then are lowered into water and asked to expel all the air from your lungs and remain motionless while your underwater weight is measured. You do this three times, and your weights are averaged.

The hydrostatic method was considered the gold standard of body fat measurement for many years, until DEXA hit the scenes. DEXA (Dual-emission X-ray absorptiometry) is used for bone-density testing and is basically an X-ray that is done while you lie still on a bed for a few minutes. I have tried this one personally, but like hydrostatic weighing, it is inconvenient (you have to find a facility that has the equipment) and costly.

The final method of testing body fat is called Bioelectrical Impedance, and it is the one you frequently see at gyms and medical facilities where you step on a scale, hold a pair of handles, and an electrical charge is sent through your body to determine your body fat percentage. This is the *least* accurate method of testing because it is highly sensitive to the subject's hydration level, which makes me wonder why it also seems to be the most widely used.

There have been studies showing that body fat calipers come very close in accuracy to the hydrostatic test, so just trust me on this and go with my recommendation. Remember, trend is your friend and really all that matters when you are grinding away trying to lose fat. Once you hit that single-digit body fat level and can show off your ripped six-pack abs, will you really care if you are half a percent more or less than you appear to be?

There's no perfect answer for how often you should weigh in and check your body fat. At a minimum I think you need to weigh in and measure body fat once a week. Many people I know who are cutting will weigh themselves every morning. Yes, like a science experiment, the greatest chance of success comes when you have as many data points as possible, but don't get too manic about it. Daily weigh-ins can cause frustration and freak-outs if the scale doesn't move. (Remember the plateaus we just talked about.) Just ensure that you're trending in the right direction, and tweak your approach accordingly.

Speaking of tweaks, we're about to cover one that I'm sure will be the consensus favorite among readers, ha! It's time to talk about cutting alcohol from your diet.

KEY TAKEAWAYS

- Every calorie is comprised of three macronutrients: protein, carbohydrates, and fat. Each macronutrient serves crucial functions within your body.

- If you know the macronutrient composition of a food item, you can use 4-4-9 to determine the number of calories it has.

- Fad diets fail because they restrict your food choices and keep your body from getting the protein, carbs, or fat it needs to function properly.

- When you adhere to the Laws of Energy Balance and Macronutrient Balance, food choice is not that important.

- You can't achieve long-term success with bad foods as a regular part of your diet.

- Junk food leaves you feeling less full because it's so dense calorically compared to clean foods. On a caloric deficit, you want to feel full.

- With *Hack Your Fitness*, you'll eat more than you're used to because you're eating natural, lean foods that are less dense calorically.

- On workout days (three times a week), protein will constitute 45 percent of your daily caloric intake, and on rest days (four times a week), protein will be 55 percent of your calories.

- On workout days, your remaining calories will be 40 percent carbs and 15 percent fat. On rest days, it's more of an even split: 20 percent carbs and 25 percent fat.

- Protein is kept high every day because it leaves you feeling satiated after eating.
- Don't listen to people who say carbs are bad or that you shouldn't eat fat. Those people are idiots. Your body needs the right combination of carbs and fat in conjunction with the proper protein intake.
- Tracking macros is easier when you front-load the work and find go-to meals.
- Find a tracking method you like and stick with it. The same goes for the website you use for your nutrition information.
- A go-to "Hacker Friendly" food list helps you front-load the legwork with macronutrients.
- Ditch supplements, and chew your calories.
- Protein shakes are only recommended when you have to hit your protein intake for the day and you're too full to eat any more food.
- Take a simple multivitamin to help with your micronutrients.
- Your weekly weight loss will be between 0.7 and 2 pounds starting out, based on your starting body fat percentage.
- Remember that weight loss is not linear. The amount of weight you start out losing the first few weeks won't be the amount you lose every week.
- Don't panic if you hit a weight loss plateau.
- Body fat calipers are the most affordable and easiest way to measure body fat.

ACTION STEPS

- Using your daily calorie budget, determine the amount of each macronutrient you need to consume on workout and rest days. Keep in mind that your calorie budget is roughly 40 percent lower on rest days compared to workout days. (Go to http://hackyour.fitness/resources to download the free Macro Calculator.)

- Buy a pair of body fat calipers and a food scale.
- Take a day and weigh lots of different foods to determine the macronutrient composition and the caloric density.
- Create your own "Hacker Friendly" meals list that you can reference easily when considering your meals for the day.
- Establish your routine—tracking, weighing, and measuring body fat—and begin practicing it to ingrain this behavior as a new habit in your life.

CHAPTER 6

YOU BOOZE, YOU LOSE: THE TRUTH ABOUT ALCOHOL

I feel sorry for people who don't drink. When they wake up in the morning, that's as good as they're going to feel all day.

— FRANK SINATRA

Yeah, so...this part of the diet is zero fun. I get that. Really, I do.

Honestly, I don't want to be the guy who says you can't drink for twelve weeks. I enjoy drinking as much as anyone. The problem many of us face is a lack of control when we drink. One beer becomes ten, one glass of wine turns into a full bottle, and a round of shots leads to you waking up in a bathtub half-naked and without your phone (or kidneys). We've all been there.

That's the reason I'm asking you not to drink for twelve weeks. I know it's a big sacrifice. I've sat across from plenty of friends whose jaws have dropped when I got to this part of the diet. Their stunned expressions would make you think I handed them a death sentence.

"You can't be serious, Jay," they stammer. "No alcohol for twelve weeks? Are you crazy?"

When I pitched this program to you, I asked for twelve weeks. In the scope of your life, that's a blip. The difference with this blip is that it can change your life. This will be a test of your commitment. If you can do everything else I'm asking of you, except stop drinking, then I don't think you're serious about this program.

If you're strong enough psychologically to cut out booze, you're absolutely going to be successful. There are not many things in life that offer this kind of guarantee. But realize that when I say no alcohol, that means literally no alcohol. Not one beer, glass of wine, or tequila shot at the bar.

It wasn't easy for me to give up drinking during my first twelve weeks. I love going out with friends and having a good time. I found strength during that time from—where else?—my wife, who was pregnant. Since she couldn't drink, I told myself I was showing solidarity with her by remaining sober. We suffered through it together.

The sacrifice grew easier to deal with over time as I saw the gains I'd been desperately seeking for years. Not being able to drink was the furthest thing from my mind. I can't promise that your desire to drink will disappear over the next twelve weeks, but I can promise that the sacrifice will be worth it in the end.

Once I explain why alcohol is a fitness hacker's kryptonite, I think you'll appreciate why I'm asking you to lay off booze for twelve weeks. You may still hate it, but at least you'll understand. To make it easier, I've kept this chapter short and sweet.

THE GOOD, THE BAD, AND THE UGLY

If it is endurable, then endure it. Stop complaining.

— MARCUS AURELIUS

We'll start with a couple pieces of good news about booze. First, alcohol you drink can't be stored as body fat, because your body is incapable of converting ethanol into a lipid that can be stored as fat. There are also some health benefits associated with alcohol. For example, studies have shown that alcohol can improve insulin sensitivity, and on average, moderate drinkers live longer than nondrinkers. That's the good news.

If alcohol can't be stored as fat and has health benefits, then why can't you drink?

The dirty secret of alcohol is that it blocks fat oxygenation. When you drink, the alcohol you just ingested takes priority in your body's metabolism. It jumps to the front of the line and highjacks your metabolism, essentially. Your body's fat-burning capability shuts off, and all your body's resources become focused on breaking down the alcohol first.

With your body's fat-burning capability switched off, anything that you eat after you booze is going straight to fat storage. It's not the calories in the alcohol that make you fat. It's all the crap you eat with it and afterward that's the problem. Those are the killer calories.

Alcohol, on the other hand, represents empty calories nutritionally. Remember the formula 4-4-9? Well, alcohol comes in at a seven on that scale. It's not a macronutrient, but it has seven calories per gram. When you're working on a caloric deficit for this program, you want to chew every calorie you have. If you drink one beer that's 150 calories, you just spent 10 percent of your calories for that day. Have a couple of drinks at the bar, and you're going to be starving the rest of the day. Are those drinks really worth it?

When consumed in large quantities, alcohol significantly lowers your testosterone level. That's a big problem since you need testosterone to build muscle. Overconsumption also has a detrimental effect on your mind when you're on a fitness program.

When you're drunk or hungover, your inhibitions are lowered, and you make bad diet decisions. We've all been there and done that. When you're drunk, late-night cravings turn into late-night food because your willpower is gone. When I'm hungover, burgers and pizza and Bloody Marys sound like amazing ideas. The sober version of Jay would never eat those foods, but hungover Jay is like, "Screw it, I have to eat this."

Alcohol also derails your workout program. I don't know if you've ever tried to work out when you're hungover, but it's brutal. Whenever I have a big night, the next morning I'm in really bad shape. Even if it was Friday when I partied, by the time Sunday comes around and I'm getting ready to do my squats, I still feel slightly off. Because I drank two days earlier, I'm going to be weaker for my next workout.

Again, is it worth it?

I think the more you become in tune with your body, the more your feel it when you drink and the more it will hamper your gains. If you're hungover, first of all, you're probably going to skip your workout. If you do manage to get your workout in, it's probably going to be a shitty one because you're not going to be feeling it and pushing yourself at max effort. By missing out on that one workout, you're basically missing out on one week of gains.

Furthermore, alcohol dehydrates you and seriously affects your water retention. It can throw your weight off, too. After a big night of drinking, your body is so dehydrated that it pulls in all the fluids you drink. This means your weight will sometimes actually be lower on the morning after. Ironically, since you're so dehydrated, the body you see in the mirror will actually look more lean.

"Damn," you'll say, admiring your reflection. "I should go drinking all the time!"

Please don't look at your reflection and say that to the mirror. You and I both know that as you rehydrate over the course of the day, you'll start retaining water again and become bloated. Whatever your data point was from that morning, throw it out!

MODELS AND BOTTLES: YOU WILL GET TO DRINK AGAIN

I don't want to get you drunk, but, ah, that's a very fine Chardonnay you're not drinking.

— PATRICK BATEMAN

That's it in terms of the positives and negatives of boozing. When it comes down to it, I just want to see if you're mentally strong enough to give up something you'll enjoy today for something you want the most. Remember that Neal Maxwell quotation from earlier? "Never give up what you want the most for what you want today."

When the twelve weeks are over and you've become adept at counting calories and tracking your macros, you'll have the flexibility for an occasional drink. There are strategies we'll get into later that let you manipulate your diet around big drinking events to provide a buffer for those empty calories. *Hack Your Fitness* isn't like Atkins where you can never have carbs again. You get to drink, and I'll teach you how to handle it right.

For me, alcohol was another great impediment to making progress because I never thought that I could give it up for a long of a period of time. When I finally did, my life changed in three months. Every piece of this diet works together like a well-oiled machine. You can't do everything else and skip one of the steps.

When you do that, the whole thing falls apart.

Now that I can drink again, I usually do it only on the weekends. I don't recommend anyone drink heavily more than once a week after the initial twelve weeks. It's not healthy to drink more often than that, and you can't forget about all those negative side effects.

Whenever you do drink after the twelve weeks, the alcoholic beverage gets logged as carbs when you're tracking your macros for the day. The empty carbs won't help your macros any, but if you're out with friends or need to blow off steam after a rough work week, you can definitely afford to indulge.

Whew! We did it. Now we can move on from the not-so-fun diet part to the section you're probably most excited about: the exercise routine.

KEY TAKEAWAYS

- Lack of control when drinking is the biggest threat to the *Hack Your Fitness* diet, not the alcohol itself.
- For the twelve weeks you're on *Hack Your Fitness*, you can't drink.
- The good news is that alcohol can't be stored as fat.
- The bad news is that booze blocks fat oxygenation and hijacks

your metabolism, meaning everything you eat *after* you drink gets stored as fat.

- Alcohol clocks in at seven calories per gram.
- Alcohol lowers your testosterone, which is needed for building muscles.
- Your decision making when you're hungover is not great. You're likely to blow off your workout and eat terrible foods the morning after.
- Even if you do work out hungover, it'll most likely be a terrible workout.
- Alcohol dehydrates you and affects your water retention, which can throw off your weight.
- Yes, you will get to drink again after the initial twelve weeks. When that time comes, limit yourself to drinking once a week.
- For macro tracking purposes, alcohol gets logged as carbs.

ACTION STEP

- Bid farewell to drinking for the next twelve weeks. You can do it!

PART THREE

—

OLD IS GOLD

CHAPTER 7

THE TACTICS OF HACKING FITNESS: COMPOUND LIFTS

Strength does not come from winning. Your struggles develop your strength. When you go through hardships and decide not to surrender, that is strength.

— ARNOLD SCHWARZENEGGER

Milo from Croton was known as the greatest wrestler in ancient Greece. He won six Olympic laurels and achieved the "Grand Slam" by winning four athletic festivals in the same cycle. He was the sixth-century-BC version of Michael Phelps, basically.

Milo achieved his legendary strength by borrowing a newborn calf and carrying it around town with him every day. As the calf grew, so did Milo's muscles because the weight that he was lifting over the same distance was growing. Even when the calf grew into a bull, Milo could lift him because his strength had increased so much.

The story of Milo and his calf demonstrates a concept called progressive overload that is foundational to *Hack Your Fitness*. The theory of progressive overload is that in order to get stronger over time, you must increase either the number of reps or the amount of weight you're using each time you work out. That's one cornerstone of this program.

Compound lifts comprise another cornerstone. Every strength and conditioning program should include the three compound lifts: squat, deadlift, and the press (also called the overhead press and not to be confused with the bench press). When Milo squatted down to lift his calf every morning, and raised it over his head at day's end to set it down, in essence he was practicing compound lifts.

Long before gyms existed, compound lifts were the exercise of choice for bodybuilders. Those beefy, mountainous men only needed barbells to achieve the look they wanted, which was far different than what we picture today. Make no mistake, these dudes were still jacked and had good definition, but their bodies just don't compare to what you see with modern bodybuilders. The human body has simply evolved with better training and nutrition. The limits of possibility for the human body have expanded.

Everything changed in the 1970s when a man named Arthur Jones introduced the world to resistance training equipment. His Nautilus machines were revolutionary, and his pitch to gyms was ingenious. By buying an entire machine set, gyms could put customers on a circuit that included twelve machines working different muscle groups in isolation. Nautilus machines required very little training, and customers didn't have to rest long between sets, since each machine worked a different part of the body. The whole circuit took thirty minutes.

You can see the appeal of these machines and circuit training if you're a gym owner. First off, these machines require little to no training, so you don't have to hire additional staff to teach clients how to use them, and the risk of injury was little to none. More appealing is the fact that a thirty-minute circuit creates a streamlined traffic flow and increases the efficiency of the exercise taking place. More traffic plus greater efficiency equals more money.

Nautilus was a huge commercial success. Within a few years, it seemed as if every gym in the United States had these machines, and circuit training came into vogue. Compound lifts—which take longer and require proper training—declined in popularity with bodybuilders, who opted for circuit training as their preferred path to isolation training. In order for their biceps to pop and their shoulders to be shredded, bodybuilders needed to hit every muscle group in isolation, and Nautilus machines allowed them to do just that.

The bodybuilding community embracing circuit training was a big deal even for the average Joes who didn't need isolation training. In the pre-Internet days, bodybuilders served as gatekeepers in the world of fitness instruction. If the man with bulging biceps and gargantuan traps prescribed you an exercise regimen, who were you to doubt it? When bodybuilders endorsed circuit training, anyone who was looking to get fit noticed.

Even today with the resurgence of compound lifts due to CrossFit and other workout regimens, most gyms have disproportionately more circuit machines than free weights. I can just see Milo having a "headdesk" moment right now.

If you want to keep your gym membership for *Hack You Fitness*, feel free. But know that you don't have to. A simple squat rack and bench setup in your basement is all you need for success. Whether you decide to go all out with a full rack setup from Rogue Fitness or go minimalist with a foldable Vulcan Rack from IronMind (in true MEFP fashion), for *Hack Your Fitness* your equipment needs will be sparse and your time commitment minimal. I've always felt that my time and money is better spent elsewhere, so I have a simple squat rack setup at home that I use.

WHY COMPOUND LIFTS BURN MORE FAT THAN CARDIO

The story of the human race is the story of men and women selling themselves short.

— ABRAHAM MASLOW

Compound lifts are key to unlocking the holy grail of fitness: body recomposition. No other workout is better for building muscle and burning fat, including cardio.

My colleagues didn't believe me when I told them as much last year. We all went out for lunch one day, and they were sitting around the table pondering how they were going to burn off the calories we were about to consume. Colleague A got the ball rolling when she told us about Tabata training and how it sets your workout intervals to music.

Not to be outdone, Colleague B told us about a "hot Singaporean dude" who does high-intensity interval training and has a hundred thousand Instagram followers. Watching his videos was her preferred workout regimen. (I'm sure his hotness in no way affected her decision.)

Colleague C joined in to sing the praises of high-intensity interval training (HIIT) and the afterburn effect that allows you to burn calories for hours after you work out. As they went on about all this, I sat there listening with slight amusement. Finally, one of them turned to me and asked, "Hey, Jay, what sort of cardio do you do?"

"I don't," I told them. "I lift heavy. I hate cardio."

My answer brought the conversation to a screeching halt. They looked at each other a little stunned. I guess my answer wasn't typical of a "fitness guy." But before I could explain myself, they went back to talking about the hot Singaporean dude on YouTube.

I found that whole conversation, and their reaction to my answer, intriguing. Here I was, stronger and leaner than I'd been in my entire life, and none of them asked me why I didn't do cardio. Not only that, but they also watched me eat more than anyone else at the table. While they nibbled on salads and fruit, I was crushing steak, a baked potato, and escargot since it was a workout day and I'd calculated my macros for the meal earlier that morning.

While I was enjoying freedom, my colleagues were saddled with the dogma that exercising is a necessary evil to offset your lifestyle. They couldn't enjoy a meal without worrying about calories, interval training, and the afterburn effect.

As I sat there, I remember feeling a true sense of control as I ate what I wanted with no guilt. I had escaped the rut they found themselves in and knew exactly where diet and exercise would take me.

My colleagues also suffered due to their mistaken belief that high-intensity interval training produces the best afterburn effect. What the layman calls the afterburn effect is actually excessive post-exercise oxygen consumption (EPOC). These are the various processes your body undertakes to recover after a strenuous workout. For reasons I've never fully understood, the afterburn effect is only ever associated with cardio sessions.

But if you compare it to everything else, does HIIT actually have the highest EPOC?

On a scale of time you spent doing steady-state cardio on an elliptical or treadmill versus time spent doing high-intensity interval training, the afterburn effect of course is greater following HIIT. That's why HIIT has become so popular in the cardio world. Thirty minutes of intense exercise punctuated by short breaks produces far better results than an hour on the bike. If you care at all about your time or your results, why wouldn't you choose HIIT?

Unless, of course, you're measuring it against compound lifts, in which case you'd see that there isn't even a comparison. The EPOC resulting from compound lifts far exceeds that of resistance circuit training, steady-state cardio, or even HIIT by a landslide. The difference is literally off the charts—up to forty-eight hours after a heavy compound lift, your body is *still* recovering.

It is scientifically proven that past the age of twenty-five, our metabolisms slow down as much as 2–4 percent every single year. That's around the same age in life when we start adding a job, family, and other obligations to our plate, all of which require increasing amounts of our precious time. From a pure time perspective, the return on investment (ROI) of compound lifts, which are proven to have the highest EPOC, is a runaway victor. When you stack everything up, it's easy to see why my MEFP includes compound lifts and nothing else.

DON'T THINK, JUST DO

Don't think about winning the SEC championship. Think about what you need to do in this drill, on this play, in this moment. That's the process. Let's think about what we can do today, the task at hand.

With *Hack Your Fitness*, you're only going to spend forty-five minutes working out three times a week. I've mentioned this already, but I don't think it gets old wrapping yourself in that wonderful truth. Gone are the dog days of one-hour workouts, six times a week, as miserable as they were.

Each of the three workout days will be dedicated to one of the main "big three" compound barbell lifts: squat for your legs, press for your shoulders and upper body, and deadlift for your back. You might have tried these exercises in the past, but we're going to perfect them as part of this program.

The *Hack Your Fitness* training program was designed to be as efficient as possible. As such, I designed the entire workout so it can be done completely with a simple barbell squat rack and bench. No more wasting time waiting on circuit training; no more waiting for machines. You get to the rack, get to work, and get out of there. That's the beauty of the MEFP.

That said, there is a degree of flexibility with the training

THE TACTICS OF HACKING FITNESS: COMPOUND LIFTS · 163

program. As hackers we need to be nimble and able to adapt to any situation that is thrown at us. In the following chapters we will go over the "big three" lifts in detail. These are the most important exercises that are paramount to your workout regimen; they are required of you at the absolute minimum. We've just gone over in length why compound barbell lifts are the best exercises in the world for you, so I'm sorry to say, the "big three" are nonnegotiable.

When it comes to the other exercises in each workout, there is some room for flexibility and substitution depending on what equipment your gym has available and how much time you have to work out. But I can say this: once you've tasted the delight and convenience of being able to do all your workouts with one squat rack and not having to roam the gym, you'll want to stick to what I prescribe.

What about using dumbbells for the "big three" lifts? Won't that improve symmetry? The short answer is no. First of all, you aren't trying to become a body builder, so who gives a shit about symmetry? Second of all, if you are truly able to build up your strength with barbell training, your symmetry will be just fine. You won't find anyone out there who can deadlift 2.5 times his body weight, squat twice his body weight, and press one times his body weight complaining about symmetry. That's the truth.

On a more serious note, training exclusively with dumbbells does have its merits as a secondary or assistance exercise *after* you've completed the "big three," but not for the main lift. There are a few reasons for this, but the main issue is that progressive overload is nearly impossible using dumbbells due to the simple fact that dumbbell increases are much harder to do as you go up in weight as opposed to increasing load on the barbell. Dumbbells make it very difficult to lift heavy because you are limited by the strength of your grip, and it is awkward to try to get the dumbbells up to the starting position. With dumbbells you basically cannot get a decent leg workout in. Finally, it is just much more time consuming to adjust weight using dumbbells compared to simply sliding another plate on each side of the barbell. Ditch the dumbbells for now, and just follow the system.

I've included a sample workout chart below that shows all the lifts you'll do each day. We'll cover the "big three" lifts in the next few pages. For information on the rest of the lifts, you can skip to the appendix or visit http://hackyour. fitness/resources, where I explain them all in detail. I've also included an exercise substitution matrix in the appendix for your easy reference in case you need to improvise.

But my recommendation is crystal clear: *If your gym does not have a squat rack you can use, go find a gym that does.*

Day 1: Squat	Sets x Reps	Set 1 @ Max	Set 2 @ 90%
Back Squat	2 x 6-8	100 x 6	90 x 7
Front Squat	2 x 6-8		
Calf Raise	2 x 10-12		

Day 2: Push	Sets x Reps	Set 1 @ Max	Set 2 @ 90%
Overhead Press	2 x 6-8		
Bench Press	2 x 6-8		
Incline Press	2 x 6-8		
Dips	2 x 6-8		

Day 3: Pull	Sets x Reps	Set 1 @ Max	Set 2 @ 90%
Deadlift	2 x 6-8		
Chin Ups	2 x 6-8		
Bent Over Row	2 x 6-8		
Shrugs	2 x 10-12		

On workout days you'll attack your lifts with intensity and focus. No chatting between sets or checking Facebook on your phone. These lifts are done at max effort, so your mind must be free of distractions. I know I'm being a stickler, but I promise—your focus makes a difference.

Compound lifts require more education than isolation machines. If you don't know anything about the barbells, you might go to the gym and be daunted by the squat rack. That's where the meatheads congregate, right? They're over there huffing and puffing and dropping weights on the floor like a bunch of animals. Who would walk over there? It's much easier and quieter to sit on an isolation machine and do your own thing.

I get that, although I will say meatheads are entirely harmless once you get to know them. In fact, you'll often find under that sweaty exterior is a kind and gracious soul willing to help you with your lifts. But it's intimidating at first, no doubt about it.

If this hurdle is tripping you up, I want to briefly explain why you shouldn't run for the safety of the isolation machines.

Isolation exercises are not as effective in strength training as compound exercises for the simple reason that the human body functions as one big system, or the sum of many parts. Your body is not made to isolate a single muscle and work it alone. That's unnatural. The central nervous system controls your muscles together in a complex way, and when you exercise your body as a whole, your body will reap the benefits.

One of those benefits is what I like to call balanced coordination. (I prefer this term to the more commonly used "core strength.") If you're under a load, whether it's a squat or an overhead press, there's a lot more going on with your body than if you're sitting on a Nautilus machine doing an isolation movement. You have to adjust your balance and coordination in order to execute those lifts, and that kind of training benefits your whole system. (Are you beginning to see why compound lifts have the highest EPOC?)

Your bones also benefit from compound lifts. As living tissue, your bones get denser the more you lift heavy. This is particularly beneficial for older trainees who spend years doing compound lifts and enjoy stronger bones as a result.

You can get all the benefits of circuit training from your compound lifts and then some. That's why old is gold, and why you shouldn't be afraid of the meatheads—they're your friends!

It might sound ridiculous after I just explained why you shouldn't be afraid to educate yourself on compound lifts, but the truth is you don't *need* perfect form for these lifts. Proper form is important, but you're not reading this book to prepare for a powerlifting competition. (If that's the case, you're reading the wrong book!) You picked up *Hack Your Fitness* to optimize this area of your life. We want to get strong and lean as quickly as possible.

Years in the gym have taught me that the human body is quite amazing. When you're stressed under a load, say a heavy squat, your body is going to automatically find the shortest path to get that bar back up to safety. Call it a survival instinct. Knowing that, I'm going to teach you just what you need to know, the basics of each main compound lift so you can avoid injuring yourself. Don't get caught up in the technicality of each one. As the section title implies, we don't want to overthink things.

Far too many fitness sites these days go too deep into the mechanics and form of each exercise and overcomplicate things. In the time it takes you to finish reading a super technical article on how to perform the perfect bicep curl, you could have gone in and completed an entire workout. Just like getting caught up in daily body-weight fluctuations, we don't want to get too manic about these lifts. We want to learn the fundamentals and then hack our way through it.

TRACK YOUR LIFTS

What's measured improves.

— PETER F. DRUCKER

Using progressive overload as part of our exercise routine means we need to track every lift that we do. Failure to do so is the one thing that will hold you back from making consistent gains in the gym. Let me state this another way. The single most important part of working out is logging in your workout. Yes, it's *that* important.

We track every lift because our success depends on having as many data points as possible. You can't track your progress without data, and you won't know if you've plateaued unless you track. If you're in the dark on how much weight or how many reps you did last week, then your workouts this week will suffer. You can't make gains unless you track. Has your progress with the squat stalled out? Maybe this week you can pump some extra effort into that lift to break out of your rut. Tracking will give you the motivation that you need to progress each and every week.

By now you know that *Hack Your Fitness* is all about efficiency, and tracking your lifts is one of the key time-saving techniques that you will employ. When you get to the gym, you will know exactly how much weight you lifted last week, and how much you need to put up this week. Don't tell yourself that you'll remember the weights and reps from one week to the next, because we both know that's a lie. Most people can't even remember what they had for breakfast this morning (I do—nothing!). By tracking you will condense your workout to include zero wasted time—a true surgical strike.

Your workout logs are a road map for the gym, providing you with valuable information about your past workouts and precious insight into your future workouts. I have a Moleskine notebook that I use to track my lifts, as you can see from the sample workout log I've included. One notebook lasts me about three years. Some people use their phone, and others use a spreadsheet. It doesn't matter which way you track; just make sure you do it.

When you look back at your notes, there's nothing sweeter than seeing your progress from week to week. We've talked about little rewards during these next twelve weeks, and I can't think of anything more gratifying than having the proof of your increased strength staring back at you from the page or screen. Trust me when I say you don't want to write down less weight or fewer reps than you did the week before. It's demoralizing.

These results can punch you in the gut or kick you in the ass. I prefer the latter.

LESS IS MORE

Work very hard on your workouts, but do as little as possible between them. Extra work will defeat your purpose.

— PERRY RADER

The foundation of this fitness program is the squat, which also happens to be the most physically demanding of our lifts. The deadlift is the second on that list, so we're going to put at least two days of rest between our squat and deadlift. Make it easy on yourself and just use my schedule for lift days: squat on Sunday, press on Tuesday, and deadlift on Thursday. I put three days between the squat and deadlift, then two days on the backside, because my body needs as much time as possible to rest and recover.

Squatting on Sunday also helps take the stress out of Monday mornings. I think we can all agree that Monday doesn't need any help in the stress department. By jump-starting your week on a Sunday and getting your most daunting workout over and done with, psychologically your week will be a breeze. You've already accomplished the most difficult physical task, and the week hasn't even started. No more Sunday night blues, and no more Monday morning scramble.

There are a couple of other reasons why I recommend a

weekend workout that may not seem intuitive to you right now, but you'll thank me later. Getting a workout in on the weekends allows you to eat big on one of your two weekend days. The benefit of this is twofold. First, psychologically it is a lot easier to manage your rest day calories during the work week when you are busy with your routine or stuck in an office environment. On weekends, human beings are naturally in more of a relaxed mental state, and with the kitchen just a few steps away at home, it is a lot harder to fight the temptations that will occur when you are on lean day calories. This is a point you won't think about right now at the beginning of a program, but as you lean down and your calorie budget gets continually slashed every week, you'll be happy to implement these advanced strategies to help you cross the finish line. The second benefit is more obvious, and that is simply the fact that most social engagements tend to occur on the weekends, so you will want to have a higher calorie budget then.

The protocol we're going to use is called reverse pyramid training (RPT). The way most people lift is they start with a warm-up and gradually work up to their max weight over the course of three to five sets. Reverse pyramid training is the opposite. Your first set (after your warm-up) is going to be your heaviest set, and then on your second set you'll reduce the weight and do more reps. You start at your max weight and work down, not the other way around.

We use RPT because it is hands down the best way to achieve the maximum amount of results in the minimum amount of time. You're training extremely hard, but not for very long. It's a fitness hacker's dream!

Your first set will be the heaviest, but you're attacking it when you're the freshest and your muscles are strongest. Psychologically, you benefit from knowing that you've done the hardest thing first (kind of like squatting on Sundays!). Even with the higher number of reps, that second set will seem a little bit easier since you've descended from the mountaintop.

You're going to do some warm-up sets so that you're not going in cold, but then on your first set, you're going to use max effort. The rep range on most of these lifts is between six and eight, which is lower than you might expect, but that's because we're lifting heavy. Finding your working weight—the weight in which your reps fall between six and eight *at max effort*—might take a couple of weeks. That's okay. Trial and error is part of this process. Now, when I say max effort, I really mean max effort. You should be pushing yourself to failure. At the end of each set you should not have a single rep left in the tank.

Let's take the squat, for example, and assume that your working weight is one hundred pounds. What this means is that you are able to do six reps at one hundred pounds, but not seven. Your first set is going to be six reps of one hundred pounds. You do that set first, and you do it once. You should rest three to five minutes between sets. Stay off your phone, and keep your mind focused on the workout. Use that time to jot down the results of the set you just did.

For the second set, drop the weight 10 percent. In this example, you would drop down to ninety pounds. For this set, you're going to do at least seven reps. If you can do more than eight reps of ninety pounds, then you know for next week that you can increase your second set weight by 2.5 pounds.

The same is true with your max weight. When you can do eight reps of one hundred pounds on your squat, bump up to 102.5 pounds next week and drop down to six reps. See how that goes. The key with progressive overload is to be always going up in either reps or weight. Increase your work in at least one of the two sets by either one rep or 2.5 pounds every single week. You must always be progressing.

Sticking with our squat example, your first set the second week should be seven reps of one hundred pounds if you did six the previous week. Did you do seven reps of ninety pounds for your second set? Shoot for eight reps of ninety pounds the second week. If you can do that, bump the weight to 92.5 pounds for the third week. Everyone's progress will look different, but you need to keep climbing up in reps until you hit eight, then increase your weight.

The changes I'm using in this example are extreme. You might stay at the same weight and number of reps for a couple of weeks. If you get stuck, keep your weight for the first set the same. Drop your weight on the second set, and increase your number of reps. As long as you're honestly giving max effort, you'll eventually break through.

You have to find that threshold where max effort literally means that on your last rep of that last set, you're pushing yourself to the point of failure. A lot of times on my last set of squat day, I'll fail and have to squat down and unload the rack onto the safety pins behind me. Failing blows, but it also means I am truly pushing myself at max effort, so I'm okay with that.

You don't want to injure yourself, but you should leave the gym with nothing left to give.

Your central nervous system is shocked every time you give max effort on heavy lifts. As a result, it's imperative that you rest on nonworkout days. Cardio will only detract from your strength gain by fatiguing your muscles. If you do a half marathon or HIIT the day after a heavy squat, you're not going to get the rest that you need, and your next deadlift session will suffer. You won't be as strong because you've not fully recovered.

In other words, once again, don't try to be a hero. With *Hack Your Fitness*, less is definitely more.

THE TOOLS OF THE TRADE

You're better off not giving the small things more time than they deserve.

— MARCUS AURELIUS

The fitness industry would have you believe that more accessories make for a better workout. But we know better, don't we? The hacker's mentality is to make do with as little equipment as possible. I subscribe to the "good enough" approach, which means you don't need a gym membership, supplements, fancy shoes, or the best gym bag. You just need the bare-bones essentials and to get your ass in the gym and get started.

Like everything, I've fallen into this trap before where I've proclaimed myself to be on a massive new health kick, only to spend two weeks searching online for the best gym bag before even stepping foot in a gym. I was wasting time and making excuses. I should have stopped worrying about the tools and invested my time in the trade. So let me give you the bare-bones essentials.

The first piece of equipment you will need is a squat rack and barbell with weights. Since we're doing compound lifts, this is a "must have" item. If your gym doesn't have a rack, you need to find a new gym, and if you don't want to join a gym, get one for your house. In Hong Kong, space is tight and everything is tiny, yet I somehow negotiated with my wife to give me a spare bedroom so I could have a squat rack there. I'm sure I'll have to pay the piper for that one later, but for now, I'll take it!

Squat racks aren't that expensive. The cost has come down significantly in recent years. You can get a decent rack for a couple hundred bucks. One company I would recommend is Iron Mind. Their foldable squat racks are built for heavy loads but can be stored in your closet when you're finished, so they're great if you have limited space.

The rack should have a spotting pin so you can drop the bar without injuring yourself. Most gyms have rubber floors, and you can drop the weight on the floor if needed, so a spotting pin is mainly for home gyms. Besides the rack and barbell with weights, you'll need a bench for the bench press.

As for your shoes, you need a pair with a non-compressible heel. Doing heavy compound lifts in Nike Airs or something similar would be like trying to lift weights on a pillow-top mattress that isn't firm. You're going to injure yourself with that kind of shoe.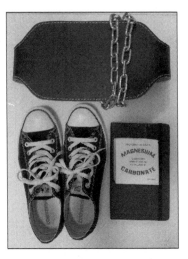

You also don't need to go out and buy a fancy pair of weight-lifting shoes. A simple pair of Converse shoes with thick rubber soles works great. That's thirty dollars out of pocket, and if you just wear them to work out, like I do, they can last up to ten years. My last pair did.

Chalk is another useful essential as you progress and start lifting heavier weights. Chalk will keep your hands dry and tight and improve your grip, particularly on your pull day exercises.

The last thing you absolutely need is a workout log. Any notebook will do, or you can use your phone. Track your weight and your reps for every lift while you're resting between sets. Don't fly blind—log your workout so you can improve week to week.

Here's something you don't need starting out: a weight-lifting belt. Don't get me wrong—these belts have their uses, especially for heavy powerlifters as the weight goes up. The belt makes a cylinder around your abs so you can squeeze harder against the belt. The problem is that most people don't know that there is actually a technique for how to use the belt, and when they put one on, they tend to think they can lift more weight than they actually can.

Here's my view: if you can't do the weight without the belt, you shouldn't be doing that weight at all. I have never used a belt and don't ever plan to. The same thing goes for wrist straps that you see people use for deadlifts since their grip is not strong enough to handle the weight they are trying to pull. ICYMI, don't try to be a hero! Learn the basics, start with a low weight, and slowly work your way up.

In case you're wondering, that belt that you see included in the photo of my tools is a dipping belt, not a weightlift-ing belt. I use this to progressively overload my dips and chin-ups because I've moved well beyond body weight for these exercises. See the appendix for a more detailed explanation of dipping belts.

The last thing you need to avoid is looking at yourself in the mirror while you lift. Most people are vain and want to watch themselves as they lift. Coming from someone whose whole program is built around vanity, I get that. But when you're squatting or deadlifting, looking in the mirror often distracts you and messes up your form. You won't need to watch yourself with this program, because your movements become muscle memory.

In fact, muscle memory is a huge injury deterrent. Once you learn the proper form in the next three chapters and practice it enough, your body will be able to execute it instinctively. When that happens, your risk of pulling a muscle due to bad form diminishes.

Proper weight is another key. Trying to lift more weight than you're capable of lifting is asking for an injury. By using our progressive overload method, you're going to progress slowly and safely up the ladder of increasing weight from week to week.

Mostly it comes down to warming up and just being smart. Give 100 percent for the hour you're working out to focus on these lifts. There's no secret to avoiding injury. The answer is simple: know your body, and don't be stupid. Stupidity will get you hurt.

On the topic of warming up, this is another area of fitness that bro scientists love to preach about in granular, excessive detail. I've read articles *about* warming up that took me ten times longer to read than my actual warm-up! There is no doubt that warming up is important, but here is my view: do the least amount of warm-up you need to feel comfortable to perform your first work set, and no more.

This will be different for everyone, but the key is to figure out what is the minimum your body needs to get "warm" and to stick with it. Don't get too bogged down in the details here. If you have no idea where to begin, here is what I suggest: do a few warm-up sets of just two reps each at 20 percent, 40 percent, 60 percent, and 80 percent of your first work set, and then get on with your damn workout. These warm-ups are quick with only one to two minutes of rest in between. You should be "warm" in five minutes and ready to go. Try it and iterate according to your needs.

Finally, check with your doctor before you start this program to make sure you're physically capable of handling such strenuous workouts, especially if you've suffered injuries in the past.

Now that you understand how your workouts are structured, we turn our attention to the finer details of lifting. First up is the foundation on which we'll build this house: the squat.

KEY TAKEAWAYS

○ The principle of progressive overload says that in order to get stronger over time, you must increase the number of reps or amount of weight you're lifting each time you work out. Progressive overload is foundational to *Hack Your Fitness*.

○ Every strength-training program should include the three main compound lifts: squat, deadlift, and overhead press.

○ Compound lifts were the exercises of choice until the 1970s when resistance training equipment (Nautilus machines) were introduced.

○ You can keep your gym membership if you want, but you don't need it for *Hack Your Fitness*. All you need is a squat rack and bench setup.

○ Compound lifts are better at burning fat and building muscle—body recomposition, the holy grail of fitness—than any other exercise.

○ Compound lifts have the highest EPOC, or afterburn effect, of any exercise. Your body is still recovering up to forty-eight hours after a lift.

○ Your metabolism slows down 2–4 percent every year past age twenty-five, right around the time you add a whole slew of new obligations. The minimal time commitment plus EPOC make compound lifts a no-brainer for the Minimum Effective Fitness Protocol.

○ Dumbbells can be used for secondary exercises, but not as a replacement for barbells during the "big three" compound lifts.

○ Isolation exercises aren't as effective as compound exercises, because the body functions as one big system, not as different muscles in isolation.

○ Compound lifts improve your balanced coordination, also known as core strength.

- You need to educate yourself on the proper technique for each lift, but you don't need to worry about having perfect form.
- The single most important thing you can do while working out is track your lifts.
- You need two days of rest between the squat and the deadlift.
- Squatting on Sundays gets your most physically demanding lift out of the way before your week even starts.
- *Hack Your Fitness* uses reverse pyramid training, or starting with your heaviest set and working down from there.
- The rep range will be between six and eight reps because you're lifting heavy.
- You might stay at the same weight and number of reps for weeks. Just keep giving max effort, and you'll eventually break through.
- On rest days, you truly need to *rest*. Your body needs time to recover.
- Besides the squat rack and bench setup, all you need for working out are shoes with a noncompressible heel (such as Converse All-Stars) and a workout log.
- Don't overthink your warm-up. Get it done quickly, and get into your workout.

ACTION STEPS

- Find a gym that has a squat rack and bench setup, or buy that equipment (plus the barbell and weights) for your house if you have room to spare.
- Buy yourself some inexpensive workout shoes, and decide how you want to track your lifts. Like everything else with this program, stick with your tracking choice.

- Commit to working out on Sundays. You'll be so thankful you did come Monday morning.
- Once you learn the proper technique in the following chapters, get ready to jump right into lifting heavy. There is no "beginner's workout" with this program.

CHAPTER 8

THE SINGLE GREATEST EXERCISE KNOWN TO MAN: THE SQUAT

The squat is a giant stimulus—not only for legs, but for other parts of the body, too. I often say that if I were thrown in jail, and I was allowed to weight train only half an hour three times a week, I would just do squats. That's it.

— DEAN TORNABENE

The squat is the single most important exercise you can do for your body, regardless of what your fitness goals are. The human body operates as a complex system, and the squat works more parts of this entire system than any other exercise.

Mark Rippetoe put it this way: "There is simply no other exercise and certainly no other machine that produces the level of central nervous system activity, improved balance and coordination, skeletal loading and bone-density enhancement, muscular stimulation and growth, connective tissue stress and strength, psychological demand and toughness, and overall systemic conditioning than the correctly performed full squat."

Essentially, Rip is saying that if you want a bigger chest, bigger arms, bigger shoulders, bigger legs, tighter abs, firmer ass, better life, then you need to do squats.

Like most worthwhile endeavors, squatting is not easy, and it certainly is not fun. I speak from experience—squatting has always been my weak point and greatest nemesis. I only started squatting seriously six years ago, because I absolutely hated working legs. You know those memes on social media where it says, "Tag someone who forgot leg day" with these huge guys who have skinny legs? That was me (only not as huge). I always skipped leg day because it was so mentally daunting.

I think my own vanity played a role, too. Like most people, I wanted to exercise parts of my body where my results would have the largest visual impact. Your legs are covered up when you go to the gym. People immediately look at your chest and your arms. That's why the bench press and bicep curls are so popular. People want their star muscles to shine.

What I didn't realize at the time was that my bicep was just a single muscle, and functionally, it does very little for your body when compared to your posterior chain (legs). To put it bluntly, my single biggest regret in fitness is that I didn't start squatting earlier. It's simply that important.

Now, let's dig into the setup for squatting.

BAR HEIGHT AND STEPPING BACK

Bar height is extremely important for these lifts. You have to set up the rack so the bar height is even with the middle of your chest. When you position yourself under the bar to squat, your knees have to be bent. A common mistake people make is having the starting rack position too high for the squat. They actually have to go up on their tiptoes to step out of the rack.

This is extremely dangerous because when you're fatigued after doing a squat, you need to be able to step forward, lean in, and rack the bar. Anything more complicated involving tiptoes is a recipe for disaster. Set the bar height at mid-chest, so when you're nearly failing on that last rep, you can easily get that bar racked.

Another important rule is to always step backward out of the rack to perform your squat, never forward. When you finish a set and you're fatigued, you want to step forward to rack the bar. At the end of your monster set at max effort, the last thing you want to be doing is looking over your shoulder trying to rack the bar behind you. This is another recipe for disaster. Always step backward out of the rack to begin your squat.

BAR PATH AND SQUAT DEPTH

The bar path is the most important component of a proper squat. We all know the shortest line between two fixed points is a straight one, so your bar path should be on a straight line. From the top of your squat to the bottom, keep the bar path as straight as possible. The more you move laterally in your squat, the less effective you will be.

The very first question people ask me when I teach them about bar path is, "What about the Smith machine?" Some gyms have what's called a Smith machine, which is essentially a squat rack with the bar path on a fixed channel. Don't use this. Your movements are more natural with a free weight squat rack than with a Smith machine. The leg press machine is also no substitute for a squat. The leg press restricts the movement of some of the joints you use, which means you won't be getting the same benefit from that exercise that you get from free weight squatting.

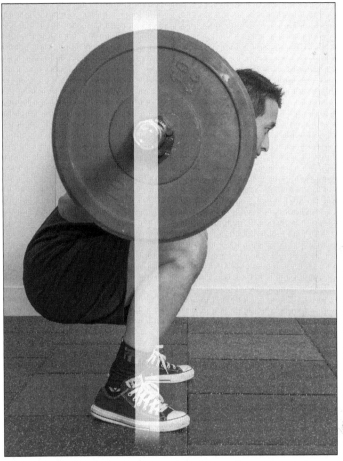

Straight Line Bar Path

The next component is squat depth. A full squat is where the hips drop below the level of the top of the knee. That's called "getting your ass in the hole." This is another common mistake I see. A lot of people load up a ton of weight but don't go down all the way. At some point in their eagerness to increase their squat, their form falls by the wayside.

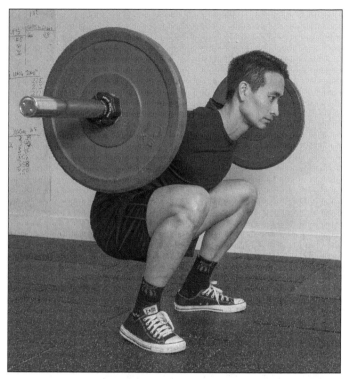

Proper Squat Depth

The only purpose this half squat serves is a great Instagram shot of how much you "claim" you can squat. It is the fitness version of the guy who pulls out all the money he has in his bank account in one-dollar bills and then "makes it rain" on social media, only to quickly redeposit the money the very next day so the check he wrote to pay his electric bill doesn't bounce.

Congratulations to those people on being able to do a half squat with more weight. It's just too bad they're not doing an actual squat. Save the stress on your knees, dip your hips below knee level, and get your ass in the hole. Anything less is a partial squat and doesn't count.

DON'T FORGET TO BREATHE

Breathing is essential for life, and that's doubly true when you're lifting. For squats, we're going to use the Valsalva maneuver. When you exert force, you want to breathe in, hold your breath, and then push. The best analogy comes from Rip himself. Picture the following situation. You're driving with a group of friends, and your car stalls out. You put the car in neutral, and everyone hops out. On the count of three, you all push the car. Someone counts, "1, 2, 3," and then...what happens? Everyone breathes in, holds it, and pushes the car together. You can almost hear the collective inhale before the push, can't you?

That's the Valsalva maneuver. Per the definition, this breathing method "increases pressure in the middle ear and the chest, as when bracing to lift heavy objects, and is used as a means of equalizing pressure in the ears." Breathe like this for every rep. Take a big breath in while standing at the top of the movement, hold on the way down, and push to get your ass out of the hole.

SQUATTING 101

I want to stress again here that you shouldn't overthink your form. When you're deep in the hole of a four-hundred-pound squat, you're not going to give a shit about your form. At that point your only concern is survival, getting your ass out of the hole, and putting the bar back onto the rack.

Rippetoe says that when you're in the hole, you should picture a chain that's linked to your tailbone. Then, imagine someone pulling that chain straight up in a vertical line and your hips coming up. The squat is actually a hip exercise, not a leg exercise. So when you go down and squat, think about getting your hips up first (out of the hole). The movement you should be visualizing is someone pulling a chain from your tailbone all the way up in a straight line toward the ceiling.

If you're new to squatting, start with just the bar. Set your feet slightly wider than shoulder width with your toes pointed out roughly thirty degrees. Make sure on the squat, when you're going down, that your knees follow out in the same path and angle that your feet are pointing. When some people squat, their knees come together or they find that their feet start curving in and they start going straight down. Make sure your knee path follows the thirty-degree angle that your feet are pointed in and that you go down all the way.

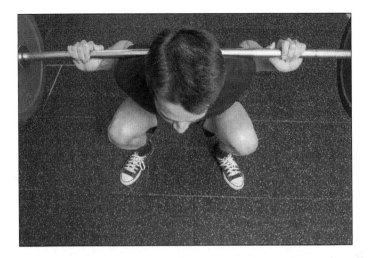

Flexibility is often an issue for people who aren't used to the squat. If you're uncomfortable squatting down in the hole, begin by practicing the squat without the bar and holding it. To improve your flexibility, sit and hold that squat stance for a long time.

When you squat, you should be looking down at the floor. Imagine a point that's ten to fifteen feet in front of you on the floor. That's where your eyes should be focused. You shouldn't be looking straight ahead at the mirror or up at the ceiling.

Okay, here we go. Step up into the rack, get under the bar, lift up, and take a few steps back. Position your feet slightly wider than shoulder length, pointed out at a thirty-degree angle. Take a deep breath in, hold it, and squat down into the hole, visualizing a vertical bar path all the way down.

Drop your hips below your knees. Your knee path should follow the direction your feet are pointed.

Now, from the bottom of the hole, you need to drive your hips up first. Don't think about pushing your legs up; focus on getting your hips out of the hole. Pull that imaginary chain up, and make sure your back is not rounded at the bottom of the squat. Go all the way up until you get back to starting position. Exhale and begin the next rep, taking a deep breath in before each rep.

Practice this form over and over again, squatting down and up, down and up. Get used to how it feels being in that deep squat. Commit it to muscle memory, and your chances of future injury will diminish significantly. When you start adding weight, your movements should be so second nature that your only concern is getting the weight up.

There's a tendency for people not to go down all the way when they add more weight (the half-squat Instagram kings). They go down in the hole and hit this threshold where, all of a sudden, fear takes over and they're unsure if they'll be able to get out of the hole. It's a pure panic moment and a squatter's biggest mental challenge. But if you have your safety pins, or your gym has rubber floors, you can dump the rack behind you with no issue. There's no reason to panic. You're safe.

Injury becomes an issue when your form is poor. Practice going down all the way until you feel comfortable doing it with added weight. Don't try to be a hero and add too much weight, because you'll most likely end up cheating on your form, thereby forfeiting that rep and leaving yourself open to injury. Be smart, and you'll be fine.

THE SEVEN DEADLY SINS OF SQUATTING

1. Starting rack position is too high: The bar should be at mid-chest level.
2. Stepping forward instead of backward *out* of the rack to begin your movement.
3. Incorrect stance, too narrow or too wide: Feet should be slightly wider than shoulder-width apart. Knees should follow the path of your feet, which should be pointing out roughly 30 degrees.
4. Not breathing properly: Learn the Valsalva maneuver.
5. Not going down deep enough: Turn off Instagram. Get your ass in the hole!
6. Not driving your hips out of the hole first: Don't push with your legs. This is not the leg press motion. Lead with your hips so they come up first.
7. Looking at your form in the mirror: Your hair looks fine. Focus on a point ten to fifteen feet in front of you.

START SQUATTING TODAY

If you weren't squatting already, stop reading this book and start practicing your squatting technique right now.

Seriously, put this book down right now. Don't make the same mistake I did and waste years of your fitness journey avoiding this essential lift. The squat is the only exercise that works your entire posterior chain, which includes the muscles in your legs and your core. Let me put it another way. If there was only one single exercise I was allowed to do for the rest of my entire life, it would be the squat.

The catch is that squatting, as I mentioned, is neither easy nor fun. All three compound lifts have such a daunting mental side to them that it's really about mind over matter. What I find that helps is, in between sets, when I'm resting those surprisingly short three to five minutes, I'm visualizing what the next set is going to look like. In my head, I'm squatting, not checking Facebook!

If you mentally run through your form during each break, then when you get up and face that next set, you'll perform it just like you rehearsed it in your mind. Roll the videotape. Don't think; just do.

We're done with the squat. The foundation for our fitness journey has been laid, and now it's time to examine the overlooked—but crucial—overhead press.

KEY TAKEAWAYS

- Your body operates as a complex system, and no exercise works more parts of that system than the squat.

- Regardless of your fitness goals, the squat is the most important exercise you can do.

- The bench press and the bicep curl are popular because of vanity, not because of their impact on your overall fitness. People want their most noticeable muscles (their chest and arms) to shine.

- When you go to squat, set the rack so the bar height is even with the middle of your chest.

- Step backward out of the rack to perform your squat, never forward.

- Your bar path as you squat should be a straight line.

- Don't bother with the Smith machine or leg press machine.

- Get your ass in the hole when you squat by dropping your hips below the level of the top of your knees.

- For all the compound lifts, breathe in at the top of your movement, hold your breath during the movement, and breathe out on your way back to the starting position. This is known as the Valsalva maneuver.

- The squat is actually a hip exercise (not a leg exercise), so when you squat, focus on getting your hips out of the hole first.

- Point your feet out thirty degrees, and make sure your knees follow that angle instead of coming together when you squat.

- When you squat, focus on a point ten to fifteen feet in front of you instead of looking at the mirror or up at the ceiling.

- While resting between sets, visualize your form for the next set.

ACTION STEPS

 If you're new to squatting, practice your form to the point where it becomes muscle memory. This will greatly reduce your risk of injury.

 Once you feel comfortable with the proper technique, put this book down, saddle up to your squat rack, and get your ass in the hole!

CHAPTER 9

THE MOST USEFUL UPPER-BODY EXERCISE THAT NOBODY DOES: THE PRESS

Compound exercises work muscles in groups. They are the most efficient way to work your muscles versus isolation/circuit training. Why spend hours in the gym hitting every body part? Compound exercises are far more effective than isolation.

— JOHN MCCALLUM

When my friends ask me what exercise I do for my upper body, I always begin with the press. The funny thing is, they automatically assume I'm talking about the bench press. But I'm not. When I explain that I'm referring to the overhead press, this is not the answer my friends like to hear. They'd rather I say "incline dumbell press" or "bicep curls" because they're interested in a big chest or big guns.

Bodybuilders established the historical precedent that each body part should be honed to peak form through isolation exercises. As we know, isolating one muscle group per lift is inefficient and not in line with the *Hack Your Fitness* mantra of "less is more." The press is useful because it works your triceps, shoulders, and upper chest all at once.

When you say "press," people like my friends assume you're talking about the bench press. The overhead press, as it's known now, used to be called the two-hand press and is actually the oldest upper-body exercise known to man that's done with a barbell. The first guy who ever worked out with a barbell picked it up off the floor and pressed it over his head. I'm guessing it was one of Milo's distant relatives.

The two-hand press fell out of favor because of the bench press, but prior to the 1950s, the two-hand press was the standard metric of upper-body strength. Bodybuilders were the ones responsible for pushing the two-hand press out the door as they switched to using the bench press to achieve a massive chest. With Arnold Schwarzenegger's chest as the ideal male physique, the bench press became so popular that it was added as a standard competition lift in the late 1960s. The final nail in the coffin was the 1972 Olympics when the two-hand press was eliminated from the weightlifting category due to difficulty in judging standards.

Since then, the bench press has been the go-to upper-body exercise.

The issue with the bench press is that you need a training partner because the movement is so dangerous when working to failure. With the overhead press, you don't need a training partner. You can do it yourself. If you fail, you just drop the weight to safety. This is why the press is the go-to upper-body lift for hackers like you and me. Curiously, hardly anyone does the press these days.

Some people do what's called a military press where they sit in a chair and lift the bar overhead, or they do a military dumbbell press where they sit on a bench and do dumbbell presses over their head.

Those are completely different exercises from the press and far inferior.

WHY SHOULD WE PRESS?

The press is the most useful upper-body exercise because you perform it standing up, which means it involves your entire body. We talked about the posterior chain in the squat chapter, and the same benefits apply here. The movement of this lift engages your legs, hips, core, chest, shoulders, and arms. It's a brutally effective full-body exercise.

The other difference is that the bench press starts from the racked position, so it's top-down. At the bottom, you see people bouncing the bar off their chest, similar to the squat where there's a little bounce. With the bench press, you can transfer your energy and use momentum to assist with the lift.

The press is more akin to the deadlift. When the motion begins, you unrack the bar at chest level. You're at a dead stop, so there's no bounce. From the bottom of the movement, you have to press the bar up without any help. That's why the press is difficult, and that's why it's the most useful upper-body workout—you're pushing yourself.

PRESSING 101

The press is a difficult move, so always start with an empty bar. You'll see guys in the gym who are able to put up two plates on the bench, three plates on the squat, four plates on the deadlift, but then they can't even do one plate per side on the press. This is likely the same reason why most guys don't do this lift—they suddenly don't look as good.

When you see guys pressing, and with proper strict form (no knee bending), it's a true metric of their upper-body strength.

If you don't know how much you can overhead press, always start with an empty bar. The bar height will be at mid-chest, same as the squat. Your grip is a bit narrower, just outside of shoulder width. Use a regular grip that includes your thumbs (some people leave those out). This lift should produce vertical forearms, meaning your elbows are tucked in and not pointing out like you have wings.

If you look like a chicken, you're doing it wrong!

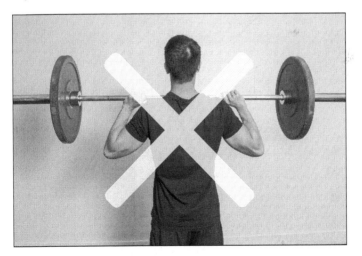

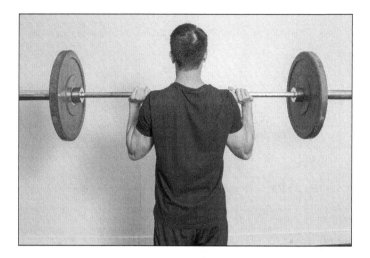

The bar should lie at the heel of your palm, not higher up where you traditionally hold the bar for other lifts. The reason for this positioning is that the amount of weight coming down during the press would put a lot of pressure on your wrists if the bar was higher in your palm. By gripping the bar in the base of your palm, that force from the bar will be transferred down the bone into your arms. A good grip saves your wrists.

Your feet should be comfortable and shoulder-width apart. I'm not a stickler on the degrees and the width of your feet on the press like I am with the squat. Lift your chest up, step into the bar, and step back from the rack. Take a deep breath, and push the bar over your head, keeping the bar path vertical. Horizontal movements limit efficiency.

Don't bend your knees for a bounce. This is the most

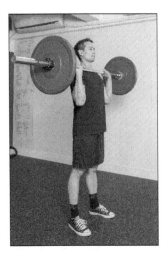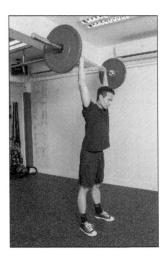

common mistake you see people make because, like the half squat, they are able to increase their weight and look better. Once they unrack the bar, they'll dip down with the knees and use that momentum to press the bar up. Unfortunately, that's a different exercise called the push press. Don't cheat when the weight goes up!

On the regular overhead press, your knees are straight. You can use a forward-and-back hip motion to get the movement started. Outside of that, there's no other movement. Keeping it strict is what ensures the maximum benefit to your upper body and shoulders.

Remember to keep the bar close to your face during the lift. The closer you keep the bar, the straighter and more efficient the bar path will be.

It took me a long time just to get up to a single plate on each side of the overhead press, whereas with other exercises, I progressed quickly. That's why I said the press is a difficult movement to learn and why most people choose to ignore it. The press might be a forgotten exercise, but I believe it's the most important upper-body lift you can do.

Now we're ready to tackle the deadlift, or as I like to call it, the most physically challenging compound lift, even more so than the dreaded squat.

KEY TAKEAWAYS

- ⊙ The overhead press (or simply the press) works your triceps, shoulders, and upper chest, making it a more useful lift than other upper-body workouts like bicep curls or the bench press.
- ⊙ The press is actually the oldest upper-body exercise involving a barbell.
- ⊙ Although the bench press is more popular than the overhead press now, it's also more dangerous and requires a training partner. The overhead press does not.
- ⊙ Like the squat, the press works your entire posterior chain.
- ⊙ If you don't know how much weight you can press, start with an empty bar.
- ⊙ Bar height should be mid-chest, your grip should be slightly wider than your shoulders, and you must keep your forearms straight. (No chicken wings!)
- ⊙ Save your wrists by gripping the bar in the base of your palm.

- Your feet should be shoulder-width apart. The angle of your feet doesn't really matter like it does with the squat.
- When you're ready, unrack the bar, take a deep breath, and push the bar straight up. Don't bend your knees for an extra bounce.
- You'll probably progress slowly on weight with the overhead press. Don't fret—this is a difficult lift.

ACTION STEP

After you squat on Sunday and rest on Monday, get back in the gym on Tuesday and try the overhead press. Don't worry if nobody else is doing this lift. They're the ones missing out on the most useful upper-body exercise you can do!

CHAPTER 10

DON'T FEAR THE DEADLIFT

Fear is good. Like self-doubt, fear is an indicator. Fear tells us what we have to do. The more scared we are working our calling, the more sure we can be that we have to do it.

— STEVEN PRESSFIELD

While it doesn't involve as much of your body as the squat, the deadlift is arguably the *most* difficult compound lift. It's so daunting that some people are scared to try it. The reason this lift inspires such dread is because the movement is performed from a dead stop. When you deadlift properly, you bring the bar down to a dead stop after each rep. (No bouncing!)

To compare, when you unrack the bar for a squat, you go down and hit a bounce at the bottom of the movement that you can use in your favor to get the bar back up. With the deadlift, you have to bend over and pull the bar up from a dead stop. There's no bounce, and gravity is fighting against you. You have to produce the force to lift the bar by yourself, and that's why the deadlift is scientifically the hardest compound exercise to do.

The deadlift is first and foremost a back exercise. Because it's the hardest lift, it's also the one that builds your back strength the best. The deadlift also counts as a leg exercise, but the squat is still far superior if you want to build your legs, and that's due to the squat depth. On a deep squat, you get down in the hole and work the entire posterior chain, whereas with a deadlift, your hips don't go down all the way to that deep pull position.

DEADLIFTING 101

The movement with the deadlift is simple—pull the bar with straight arms from a dead stop off the floor, up the path of the legs, until you're standing straight upright. You'll learn this movement quicker than you will the squat, but I would offer a word of caution: don't increase your weight too rapidly. Slow and steady increases are the key to avoiding injury, even if you master the movement easily. Don't get ahead of yourself or try to be a hero.

Remember: The deadlift is easy to learn, but difficult to execute correctly.

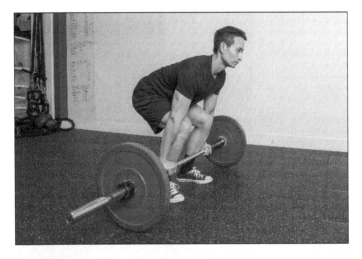

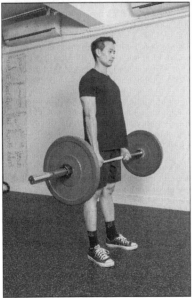

Now for the mechanics, we start with the feet eight to twelve inches apart. This is narrower than the squat stance, but your toes are at the same thirty-degree angle pointing out. When it comes up, the middle of the bar should be centered between your feet.

The bar should also be as close to your shins as possible when it comes up. If you're looking at your profile, the path of least resistance is the bar going up in a straight line. We discussed in the squat chapter that a straight bar path eliminates wasted movement. In this case, that means dragging the bar up close to your shins.

If you watch the CrossFit games, you'll notice some of the athletes wear shin guards. You can imagine why that's the case. These athletes are practicing their form so frequently that they're bound to screw up one or two reps and bloody up their shins.

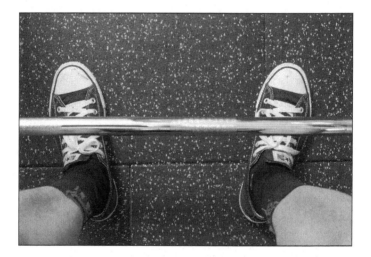

Thankfully we're not worried about perfect form or performing as many reps per week as those guys and gals. To keep your shins safe, I want you to step up to the bar and look down at your feet. Look at the distance from the back of your heel to the tip of your big toe, and envision a line cutting horizontally across the middle of that distance. That's your bar path. It's a safe distance from your shins while still being efficient.

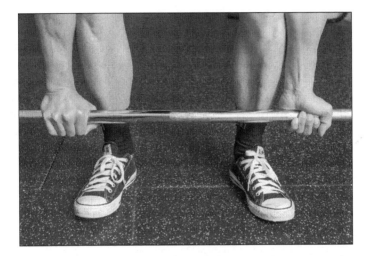

When you bend down and take a grip on the bar, your hands should be positioned just on the outside of your legs. Don't make the mistake of using a wide grip, because that's part of a different lift, one with wide legs and a wide grip called a sumo deadlift.

The most important thing to remember when you bend over to grab the bar is to do it with a neutral spine, or straight back. Don't hunch over or round your spine when you pick up the bar. Rounding your spine up or down on a deadlift is extremely dangerous and could lead to serious injury.

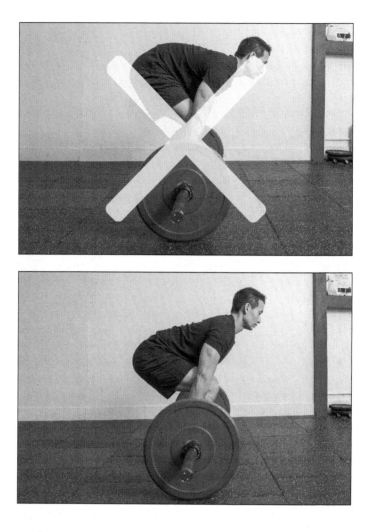

As the weight goes up, you must remain disciplined about keeping a neutral spine. Don't sacrifice form for the sake of pulling more weight.

Your hips, as previously mentioned, don't go down as far as they do on squats. The depth we're looking for here is like a half squat. Your knees will shove out when you step up to the bar because you're trying to keep the bar as close to your shins as possible.

When you begin the movement, use the Valsalva maneuver. Squeeze your chest and keep your back as straight as possible as you pull the bar up from the floor to the lockout position, which means you're standing upright. Your chest should lead before your hips in order to maintain that neutral spine and not round your back up or down.

At the top of lockout, don't hyperextend your back, don't thrust your hips forward, and don't shrug your shoulders. These are all common mistakes. For this lift, your arms are just devices that clamp onto the bar. Use your lower back and your hips to pull the bar up, not your arms. Grip strength is important for the deadlift, but this is not an arm exercise. (Chalk really helps here.)

Don't drop the bar once you get to the top of the movement. You come down the exact same way, just a little faster since there's a lot of weight coming down. At the bottom of the rep, when you've gone up to lockout and come back down, it's crucial that the bar comes to a dead stop. Starting each rep from a complete stop puts the "dead" in deadlift.

Oftentimes you'll see people bouncing at the bottom of a rep, using the inertia off the floor to cheat on the first portion of the deadlift. Bouncing makes it easy to do more reps, but you're skipping the hardest part of the lift, which is getting that bar off the floor from a dead stop. Don't cheat yourself—come to a complete stop, relax, breathe out, and repeat.

Mark Rippetoe has a wise word about the deadlift: "If a bounce is incorporated into all the reps of a set of deadlifts except the first one, much of the value of doing them is lost."

FIVE COMMON DEADLIFT MISTAKES

1. Rounding your lower back during the movement.

If you're new to deadlifting, the allure of pulling up as much weight as possible is difficult to resist because you want to look legit in the gym. I'm obviously guilty of overdoing it myself. I've hit the gym eager to set a new personal record and injured myself in the process. Speaking from experience, injuring yourself is way more embarrassing than lifting heavy weights is cool. Good form and consistent gains are your primary objectives.

2. Looking at the mirror or looking up at the ceiling.

Just like with the squat, you want to focus on a position on the floor about ten to twelve feet in front of you.

Resist the urge to look in the mirror and ogle your form.

3. Pulling with your arms, shrugging your shoulders, or hyperextending your back at lockout.

Don't give in to the desire to pull the bar up with your arms. I know it feels weird to just let them hang there, but for the deadlift, they're just functioning as clamps. There is also no need for shrugs or a hyperextension of your back at the top.

4. Using gloves or straps.

You can't use gloves, because that will skew everything you do. I suggest using chalk because it keeps your hands dry and you'll be able to pull more weight. If you have sweaty palms, the bar's going to slip out of your hands.

As your weight goes up and your grip gets weaker, you'll use an alternate grip that is similar to gripping a baseball bat, but with your hands spread out. The palm of your dominant hand (for me, my right hand) is palm down, while the less dominant (my left hand) palm faces up. You'll be able to pull more weight using the alternate grip.

5. Bouncing at the bottom and not coming to a dead stop.

I couldn't resist. I had to reiterate this one last time because that's how important I feel it is and how often I see people making this mistake. Don't be like them. You are better than that. Don't be ordinary. Be extraordinary.

MAINTENANCE: THE FINAL FRONTIER

I'm not high maintenance, you just have low standards.

— ANONYMOUS

We've reached the end of the compound lifts. Can you believe it? I can picture you in the gym making gains already. Your form is impeccable. You must've had a good teacher!

Now it's time to look at what happens after the twelve weeks are over and you've gotten control of your diet and exercise. Remember, most lifestyle changes fall apart after the goal has been reached and the maintenance phase begins.

Some of you might be more nervous about maintaining your new look than actually achieving. Twelve weeks is easy to envision, whereas the rest of your life is, well, harder to wrap your mind around. I totally understand your concerns.

Think back over my background. I'm just a desk jockey with no fancy fitness certifications to my name. This is not my profession, and I wouldn't even claim to be a hardcore fitness fanatic. The truth is, I merely designed a lifestyle program to minimize the amount of time I had to spend worrying about diet and exercise. For years, I fought against what I thought was a slow metabolism but was actually a syntax error.

All that to say: I'm just like you, and I've maintained my results for over three years now. Have I stumbled along the way, dealt with unexpected meals, drank too much on a Saturday, and felt a lacking motivation some mornings? Absolutely.

However, I've conquered them all and kept my six-pack intact. Let me show you how.

KEY TAKEAWAYS

- People are daunted by the difficulty of the deadlift because the movement is performed from a dead stop.
- The deadlift is scientifically the hardest compound lift because you have to produce the force to lift the bar by yourself.
- The deadlift is first and foremost a back exercise, although it also benefits your legs.
- The deadlift movement is simple: pull the bar with straight arms up the path of your legs until you're standing upright.
- Although the movement is easy to learn, don't be a hero and add too much weight too quickly. That's a recipe for injury.

- For your stance, keep your feet eight to twelve inches apart, toes pointing out thirty degrees, with the middle of the bar centered between your feet.

- When the bar comes up, it should be as close to your shins as possible without risking injury. If you look at your foot from heel to toes, draw a horizontal line in the middle, and that is your bar starting position.

- The width of your grip should be just outside your legs.

- When you bend down to grab the bar, keep your back straight. Curving your spine during the deadlift could cause serious injury.

- The ideal hip depth for the deadlift is about half the depth of a squat, and your knees should shove out when you reach down for the bar.

- As always, don't forget to use the Valsalva maneuver during this lift.

- At the top of your movement, when you're standing up straight, don't hyperextend your back, thrust your hips forward, or shrug your shoulders.

- This is not an arm exercise—use your back and hips to pull the bar up. Your arms are simply clamps to hold the bar.

- When you come down from the lockout (upright) position, the bar must come to a dead stop at the bottom of your movement. (Hence, the *deadlift!*)

- Don't bounce at the bottom of your movement!

ACTION STEP

After you press on Tuesday and rest on Wednesday, get back in the gym on Thursday and give the deadlift a go. Remember, safety first with this one.

PART FOUR

—

WELCOME TO THE GOOD LIFE

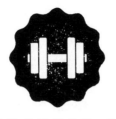

CHAPTER 11

THE ART OF FLEXIBILITY AND MAINTENANCE

Life begins at the end of your comfort zone.

— NEALE DONALD WALSCH

When doubt comes—and trust me, it will come during these next twelve weeks—or you're worried about a lack of results, the most important rule is don't panic. Don't make the same mistake I did and start changing the variables in this formula. Trust the system. The more variables you change during these twelve weeks, the worse off you'll be.

Give yourself two weeks before you change anything, and even then, only change one variable at a time. This is like a science experiment. When progress stalls, the first reaction people have is to blame the system.

"Hack Your Fitness is not working!" they shout.

Instead of doing that, the first thing you really need to do is question yourself. Are you in complete compliance with your diet? I mean 100 percent compliance. Calorie counting and macro tracking gets tedious, and after a few weeks people suddenly think they can magically eyeball the weight of food and try to wing it. Don't be lazy here. Don't let all the effort you've put in every single day go to waste.

Are you disciplined with your fasting, counting your calories, and getting the proper percentage of your macros? Are you giving max effort with your workouts? I mean truly max effort to failure?

Nine times out of ten, there is some failure in one of the areas mentioned above that is causing your progress to stall. If the answer to all these questions is truly yes, and you still haven't seen any fat loss after two weeks, then we need to take a closer look to determine what's going on.

The first thing to look at is your total daily energy expenditure (TDEE). As your weight drops, so do your calorie needs. A lot of people don't realize this, and they're still calculating their caloric intake based off their starting weight. As you lose weight, you have to adjust this number down. That's why it's increasingly more difficult to be on a caloric deficit as your weight goes down.

I suggest redoing your TDEE and macros every two weeks and running your calories based on your new weight. Your macronutrient composition will change slightly week to week. Your caloric intake will slowly go down.

The second point to keep in mind is that weight loss on the scale might be misleading since you're going through body recomposition. If you're not used to lifting weights, you'll be gaining a significant amount of muscle mass that might offset your fat loss. The key here is to focus on the visual impact if the scale isn't showing results.

The best way to measure that visual impact is with weekly progress pictures. You're the one looking at yourself in the mirror every day, which means you know your body better than anyone else. If you're taking progress pictures, you'll know whether you look leaner or fatter. Even if the scale tells a different story, your body won't lie to you.

You also shouldn't stress if your weight doesn't go down like you expect, because fat loss is what we care about, not weight loss. If your fat is being replaced with muscle, you might not weigh any less (you might even weigh more), but you're definitely losing body fat, which is the goal of this system: six-pack abs and single-digit body fat for life.

You might be tempted to do something stupid like twice-a-day cardio to jump-start your weight loss. Don't be like me and make this mistake. You're in a caloric deficit, and you're lifting heavy three times a week. You need the other four days to rest. If you add in cardio or high-intensity interval training, you're only going to burn yourself out.

Finally, I am so confident in the system that if you truly are following *Hack Your Fitness* to the letter, with 100 percent compliance in every aspect of the program, and your progress still stalls after four weeks, feel free to drop me a line at jay@hackyour.fitness and ask me anything. I will personally offer my assistance to help you out.

ADVANCED STRATEGIES: FROM LEAN TO SHREDDED

If it was easy, you would have already achieved the change you seek.

— SETH GODIN

The human body is smart. When you get down to low levels of body fat, your body tends to cling to that fat as a survival mechanism. Don't be dismayed if you hit a wall at 10 percent body fat and feel as if you can't get over it. Shedding the last bit of body fat to get into single digits is the most challenging part of this whole journey. That's why a lot of people will never achieve it. You will get there. You *will* get there.

When you're eating less and losing fat, your body's metabolism goes through adaptive thermogenesis, which is a fancy way of saying your metabolism slows down. Adaptive thermogenesis is the reason the last ten pounds are harder to lose than the first ten. Your body is fighting against you to preserve your stored fat, but there are strategies you can use to get over the hump and finally achieve single-digit body fat.

The first thing you need to do is check your diet. There's a strange phenomenon that occurs the closer people get to the twelve-week finish line. Let's say you're eight weeks into the program, you've lost a significant amount of body fat, you're looking lean and starting to see some upper abs—in other words, you're feeling great. At this point, human nature will kick in and, for whatever weird psychological reason, people will start slacking on their diet. The closer you get to your goal, the more lax you get until eventually you're outright cheating yourself.

I'm guilty of this self-sabotage, too, but I've polled friends who've done different types of workouts and diets, and they all say the same thing: the more progress you make, the more you feel like you deserve to cheat on your diet.

As you get closer to your target, you need to be more strict on your diet, not less.

You can't wing it during the home stretch. You've not reached the mountaintop after eight weeks. You haven't earned the right to coast to the finish line. The only way your numbers will keep going down is if you remain committed and disciplined.

For 90 percent of the people struggling to hit single digits, home-stretch laziness is the issue. They throw in a few extra cheat items, enjoy a night of boozing, and end up never being able to hit their goal. Don't let this become your reality. Be honest with yourself, and attack your diet harder than ever as you approach your goal. Success is sweeter than a cheat meal.

If your diet is in order, calories are in check, macros are super tight, and you're lifting at max effort to failure every single workout, and you *still* find yourself stuck, this is where I'd recommend strategic cardio. I know, I know—I've preached against cardio the entire book so far, but this is an advanced strategy for when you're doing everything else right and you're still stuck. Most people on this program won't need to do a single minute of cardio to reach their goals. I never did, and neither did any of the people I've coached. But a very small minority may need to employ it strategically to get over the hump. The key is successfully integrating cardio into your lifting schedule.

As discussed in the intermittent fasting chapter, there are two times during the day when your body is primed for fat burning. The first time is after a twelve-to-sixteen-hour fast, when the only fuel your body has left to burn is body fat. On a rest day, if you mix in some cardio after a fast, you're almost guaranteed to be burning straight body fat at that point.

The second time your body is primed for fat burning is after a heavy lift when your fuel tank is basically empty. If you throw in half an hour of HIIT cardio after you lift, you'll once again be burning straight body fat since your heavy lift depleted your body's other sources of energy.

A final strategy I recommend is called "The Regroup." After a period of prolonged caloric restriction, say eight to ten weeks, your willpower might be worn down. Operating on a caloric deficit for a prolonged period of time is both physically and psychologically draining. Most of the people who decide to wing it the last few weeks are just mentally exhausted.

I've been there and understand the strain this places on you mentally. What we're going to do is implement a cheat meal to reset your metabolism. Bodybuilders use a similar strategy when they're trying to bulk up and cut down—they eat clean all week and have one cheat day where they go nuts. I advocate a more sensible approach to cheating.

Don't go out and have a twenty-four-hour booze fest. Instead, enjoy a nice dinner where you don't have to worry with tracking. Hit the buffet if you want. For that one meal, go nuts. You're using this meal as a time to reset your body and your mind. It helps to give yourself a break mentally, and physiologically a cheat meal tricks your body into thinking you're back up to a high-calorie budget, which then kick-starts fat burning again.

After your cheat meal, you must jump right back onto the program and break through the plateau.

MAINTENANCE AND BEYOND

I am unstoppable because I decided I am.

— TONY ROBBINS

At this point, all I have to say is, "Congratulations!"

You've reached your body fat percentage goal and can now

enjoy a bit of flexibility with your diet. Now that you're no longer on a fat-burning regimen, it's time to transition to maintenance and begin adding calories back into your dietary budget.

The easiest way to do this is to recalculate your TDEE based on your ending weight. Your daily calorie budget is now equal to your TDEE. You've been on a severe caloric deficit for twelve weeks, and now you've got a couple thousand calories to add to your weekly budget. Isn't maintenance great?

There are two ways to add your calories back, and although I recommend the first one, people have seen success with both. With the first approach, you start by adding calories back to your rest days since those are the hardest days, both physiologically and psychologically, to get through with the calories being so low. Increase calories on your rest days equally.

Once you've done that, you want to scatter them over your workout days as evenly as you can. If you want to save more calories for squat day than press day, go for it.

The second way some people add back their calories is they stockpile them on Friday, Saturday, and Sunday. They stack their weekends for social reasons—big dinners with family, drinking with friends, or watching football and eating snacks. With this approach, you stick to lower calorie amounts on weekdays and splurge on weekends.

The reason I don't advocate this method is because things could potentially spiral out of control on weekends. Alcohol can impair your judgment, and societal pressures might cause you to slip up and eat two pieces of cake instead of one. But if you're fully confident you won't go overboard and overspend, by all means give it a shot.

If you're unsure which method to use, you can experiment a bit and see what works. The key here is self-awareness. I know if I used the second method I would fall off the wagon and go nuts on the weekends, so I evenly distribute my calories. You've got to know your own triggers and weaknesses during this redistribution process. At the end of the day, you only have to answer to yourself in the mirror. Just remember that.

You have to always respect the calorie budget and macros. I said at the outset that this program is a lifestyle change, which means if you want to keep the body you just worked twelve weeks for, you must stay within the calories that your TDEE dictates. Don't undo your hard work by having a bunch of cheat meals in a row or vastly altering your macros.

I've laid out the framework for how you should build your meals going forward. The macronutrient percentages aren't thrown out the window after the twelve weeks. You can't eat less protein or shift all your calories to carbs. You have to keep your protein intake high in order to keep working out and building muscle. *Hack Your Fitness* is not a quick-fix program where you get to bounce back to your old eating habits at the end. If you want a six-pack and single-digit body fat for life, a lifestyle change is the only way to get there.

Although this program helps you achieve the holy grail of fitness—body recomposition, where you're burning fat and building muscle at the same time, at least initially—some of you might be interested in bulking up rather than getting lean. My advice is, if you want to bulk, you first need to lean down to single-digit body fat before you begin your bulk.

The reason I recommend this approach is because it's more efficient to track your bulking progress if you're lean. If you're lean and you start building muscle, you'll be able to track progress easier than if you have 20 percent body fat and your new muscle is covered in a layer of fat. You're not going to be able to gauge how you look aesthetically.

Bulking is very similar to cutting under my program. You calculate your TDEE, and instead of subtracting the calories equal to one pound of body fat, you add the calories to your weekly budget. Just make sure you cut first, then bulk later.

WHEN LIFE GETS IN THE WAY: EXCESS IN MODERATION

The size of your success is determined by the size of your belief.

— DAVID SCHWARTZ

Eating is one of the greatest joys in life. You are not unique if you think food is your weakness. I can't tell you how many clients have tried to explain to me that they're the exception, that no one struggles with the desire to eat like they do.

Puh-lease.

Seriously? Who doesn't like to eat? With this program, eating is about making the right decisions for your body, not for your cravings. If everyone loves to eat, our job is to learn how to manage that love in a way that's sustainable. *Hack Your Fitness* could never succeed long-term if it robbed you of the freedom to choose what you eat.

Once you get through the twelve weeks and you've achieved your goal, you'll be armed with the knowledge to successfully navigate any situation life throws your way, whether it be a big family meal like Thanksgiving, or a hotel that doesn't have an adequate gym setup. Life happens sometimes. Situations like these might knock you off track, but if you use the strategies I'm about to lay out, you won't derail completely when life gets in the way.

Only after I designed this program was I finally able to enjoy the freedom I'd been seeking for the entirety of my fitness journey. Before I hacked fitness, there was always a certain level of guilt associated with my social activities. Every time I was out for dinner or happy hour, there was a constant battle going on in my mind.

"I'm the fitness guy. I've gotta practice what I preach."

"Should I have another drink? It's only 150 calories. That's not too bad, right?"

"You know what would go good with this buzz? A slice of pizza!"

"No! I can't have pizza. That would completely blow through my calorie budget for the day."

"Screw it, I'm getting pizza."

"I've got the number pulled up. Should I dial it? I shouldn't. Pizza is bad."

"Damn, this pizza is delicious."

I spent every night out knowing I'd have to pay penance for my sins. Dread would tie up my stomach in knots as I thought about burning off all the calories on the treadmill the next day in the gym. I was enslaved to this mentality for over a decade. I was never truly free.

Now when I go out and have a drinking session or a big meal, I do it 100 percent guilt-free. Life is so much more enjoyable when you can actually go out to eat guilt-free, knowing your big night is not going to have a detrimental effect on your fitness.

If an innocent bystander saw me eating like a maniac at my friend's birthday dinner, he or she would probably think I'm a genetic freak. No fitness guy in his right mind would be out here throwing back drinks, eating ice cream, or crushing a huge steak. I might not practice what I preach for that one single meal, but my fitness level will not change, because I'm strict with my diet otherwise and I did my homework and prep work well before the night out on the town. My actions are all premeditated with the help of calculated cheating.

CALCULATED CHEATING

Spectacular achievement is always preceded by spectacular preparation.

– ROBERT H. SCHULLER

For me, every night out and every social situation is calculated. I have my calorie budget for the week, and within that budget, I have some flexibility to manipulate those calories and prepare in advance. I go out socially about once every two weeks, and when I do, I have a system in place that allows me to have fun and maintain my physique.

Here's how it works. Let's say your best friend's birthday dinner is on Thursday night. The first thing you do is to save some of your calories for that day. Nothing extreme, maybe one hundred calories a day on Tuesday and Wednesday. You don't have to starve yourself the whole week to be able to afford yourself a higher calorie allotment for that special day.

What you're trying to offset is the poor macronutrient composition of the foods you eat when you're out. Restaurant foods are much higher in fat than you think. As we now know, fat is the densest macronutrient and the hardest to manage. You'll notice this once you're a few weeks into the program. The bread in your basket will be buttered already, or your salad dressing will be fatty, or the vegetables you order (hoping to be healthy) come out tasting like they've been stir-fried in oil. When you're trying to manage your diet, you become acutely aware of how challenging it is to eat healthy when you're out.

The biggest challenge for Thursday will be getting enough protein. Meat always costs the most when you go out, so you'll want to get all your lean protein in leading up to the big event on Thursday. The ideal setup for a social event is when it falls on a workout day, when you have a higher calorie budget anyway. When you add in those extra calories, that gives you even more buffer for the big meal. Lucky for you, Thursday is deadlift day! Don't worry, if the stars don't align, just shift your workout day that week to fall in line with the social event. It's a simple fix.

After you lift, you want to eat about 90 percent of the lean protein you need for that day with some complex carbs like veggies for lunch. Now when you get to dinner, you don't have to worry about getting your protein. You've saved most of your carbs and fat for the second meal, which is good considering what we know about restaurant food.

With the extra calories in your budget, you can now enjoy a big meal without blowing up your calorie budget or worrying about your macros. You could eat zero protein at dinner and still be fine for that day since you're only leaving 10 percent of your protein needs for dinner.

Another advantage of having a big meal on a workout day is being able to drink without worrying about working out the next morning. In the alcohol chapter, we discussed how a night of drinking completely derails your workout the next day. Since you've already done your workout, you can relax that night and have a few drinks. The next day, you get to sleep in and just rest.

A final tactic that I recommend is one called "pre-eating." If you don't feel like pounding six dry chicken breasts at lunch to get in 90 percent of your protein for the day, split it up into two meals, and have a high protein meal right before the main event. Eat lots of lean protein with some complex carbohydrates in the form of veggies. You'll hit your protein requirement for the day and show up to the main event full and less likely to go overboard.

But what happens if your social event falls on a rest day and you just cannot shift your workout to fall in line?

When this happens, you have two options: you can bump calories to that day and get your protein in beforehand (with the downside being that you have less flexibility than a workout day since your calorie budget is lower), or you can take the second, more advanced, option: an "event hacker" strategy.

Rather than eating lunch the day of your event, you follow Brad Pilon's fasting protocol for just that day and fast up until the big meal. This happens to me often when my friends want to get drinks on a Friday night. I'll deadlift Thursday morning and eat a big dinner that night. Then, instead of fasting until lunch Friday, I'll fast from Thursday dinner to Friday dinner.

The event hacker strategy is more challenging, but you do get to use all your calories for the rest day on your social event. Whatever approach you take, don't work out and then try to fast for twenty-four hours. That's just dumb. After a workout, your body needs nutrition. Either work out, eat dinner, and then fast for twenty-four hours, or stockpile calories and front-load your protein in the hours leading up to the event. Any other approach is ill-advised.

All this preparation is meaningless unless you remember an important rule: have fun! You've worked hard to obtain this physique and live a life where you can actually go out and enjoy social events guilt-free. When you do the calculations and prep work beforehand, you can use calculated cheating to enjoy the occasional splurge meal. You've earned the right to eat, have fun, and not stress out over a big meal. You've truly found freedom in fitness.

The most important thing to do on the day after a big event is to bounce right back into your clean diet. It's difficult to resist the temptation of having a greasy burger, a Bloody Mary, or a slice of pizza when you're hungover. But the faster you jump back into the program, the less detrimental the effect of that big night will be on your fat storage.

You see, fat is like muscle in that there is a maximum amount that the human body can create in any given twenty-four-hour period.

If you're able to clean up your diet the day after your event, you'll see little to no fat gain as a result of your cheat meal or drinks. It won't even be a blip on your radar.

If you indulge the day after and eat that greasy burger and drink that hair of the dog, now you're looking at two days of fat gain, which is going to set you back the rest of the week. Avoid this like the plague. You've had your fun the night before, and now it's time to get back to business.

You know what helps me when I'm hungover? I can't believe I'm saying it again, but cardio the day after really gets me back on track. A light cardio session when I'm hungover sobers me up as I sweat out the alcohol. I always feel more levelheaded afterward, and it definitely wards off any temptations of wanting to eat shitty food.

If you stick to these strategies, you'll find success in maintaining single-digit body fat for life. Once again, self-awareness is key. You have to know your body and understand its limits so you can enjoy life without squandering all your hard work.

CURVEBALLS AND EFF-UPS

A failure is a man who has blundered but is not able to cash in on the experience.

— ORVILLE HUBBARD

Unfortunately, life doesn't always respect your planning and preparation, does it? Dealing with the curveballs life throws you is another aspect of maintenance that takes practice.

Breakfast meetings are a great example of a potential stumbling block. Since I've been on IF for over six years now, I never actually get hungry for breakfast. That said, I realize breakfast meetings are a big part of the business world, and some of you might have to deal with them. There's a simple way I've found to avoid eating at these meetings.

I'll have a black coffee with me, and when someone asks if I'd like anything to eat, I politely tell them, "I ate breakfast at home with my kids" or "I'm not hungry at breakfast." I don't have to explain myself, and neither do you. If you want to offer an explanation, just tell them you're on an intermittent fasting program. You can decide if that's appropriate for the business setting you're in, but you don't have to justify anything.

There are other situations where it would be rude not to eat, such as if you're in another country and not eating is a cultural no-no. If eating is unavoidable, don't stress. One meal is not going to derail you. You can still stick to your calories for the day and hit your macros. Remember that the Law of Energy Balance supersedes all in your fitness journey. The next day, you resume intermittent fasting.

If you're in a position where you constantly have breakfast meetings, you need to shift your fasting window. Unfortunately, you can't actually have breakfast and try to follow a breakfast-skipping IF protocol, too. In order to make it work, you have to start your fast earlier. If your breakfast meetings start at 9:00 a.m., you'll have your last meal at 4:00 or 5:00 p.m. the day before and then begin your fast.

As long as you fast sixteen hours and feed for eight, your window can be moved around.

Let's talk about the challenges of travel. I love to travel for vacation, but being on the road takes me away from my home gym and messes with my routine. I take inspiration from watching my friend Darryl O'Young, the race car driver who beta tested my program and wrote the foreword for this book. He's on the road thirty to forty weeks a year traveling all over the world for different races. During his *Hack Your Fitness* journey, he was on the road an astonishing nine out of the twelve weeks of the program. He's made it work, which means you can make it work, too. Travel requires extra dedication and preplanning, but it's not impossible.

The resurgent popularity of the fitness movement means there are now few places you could travel to in the world where you wouldn't have a grocery store or a gym nearby. If your hotel doesn't have one, there's usually a gym near it that you can access.

When you have to travel for work, look up the hotel ahead of time and call about their gym. If it doesn't have what you need, look for a gym near your hotel where you can get a free trial or a free guest pass for a day. I've even gone to a gym when they're not holding classes and asked if I could test out their squat rack. If you're nice, they'll usually allow it.

For whatever reason, if you can't find a proper squat rack to use, just stick to your rest day calories and hit your macros for the duration of the trip. I think you'd have to be on a safari somewhere in Africa to have zero squat racks accessible, but stranger things have happened. Don't worry about your workouts that week. Be disciplined on your diet, and you'll be fine.

Studies have shown that giving your body one week of rest a year is beneficial if you're working out consistently every week. So as long as you're not trekking to the Arctic or cave diving twice a month, skipping one week of lifts won't hurt you.

I've made the mistake of trying to replace my usual workouts with a big cardio session to help with my calories. You can probably guess how that ended for me...not well. I'm embarrassed to say I actually injured myself when I was in San Francisco recently for a tech conference. I wasn't used to running on a treadmill, tried to do it anyway, and sprained my ankle. The injury set me back in my workouts as I waited for it to heal.

It sounds ridiculous, but it's true. If you're not used to doing a certain exercise, don't try to be a hero and jump into it on your rest week. An injury is far worse than a week off.

Don't bother with a half workout with light dumbbells,

either. You're just wasting your time and skewing how you think about your calories. You'll ask yourself, "If it's not a full workout, do I still get to eat as many calories as a workout day?" If your trip lasts less than ten days, at worst you'll lose a week's worth of progress.

Don't stress about it. Do you best when you're traveling, and you'll be fine.

We all have those days when we're pressed for time. Even if you're getting up early to work out, there will be days when life happens and you only have twenty to thirty minutes for your workout. If time is short, focus on your big lift for that day. If you can throw in a couple of other exercises, do it. If you can't, just do a kickass job with your main lift.

I always get questions about ab exercises and curls. Here's the thing: with *Hack Your Fitness*, you're going to have that six-pack and single-digit body fat. You're going to look good. If you insist on doing additional workouts to further hone your abs and biceps, that's your prerogative. The MEFP doesn't require these extra exercises.

The golden rule with any additional exercises is don't stress your core to the point where you can't do a proper squat the next day. If you want biceps like Arnold Schwarzenegger and have the time to add isolation bicep curls, go for it. Just keep yourself fresh for the core lifts, and you won't run into any problems with maintaining your gains.

THERE IS MORE TO LIFE THAN FITNESS

Now I, I go for mine, I got to shine, now throw your hands up in the sky...

— KANYE WEST

Congratulations! You are now armed with the knowledge and tools that you need to maintain the high level of fitness that you've always dreamed of.

Most of us are busy working around the clock, balancing family life, and desperately trying to make time for the gym. Not anymore. You don't need a lifelong journey to discover the secrets of fitness. *Hack Your Fitness* is your road map to success.

Like anything good in your life, you would be remiss not to share this program with anyone who has similar fitness goals as you. Anyone with the discipline and vision you demonstrated over these twelve weeks can hack their fitness to achieve and maintain single-digit body fat by spending only three hours in the gym a week. As you know, an expensive personal trainer and fancy supplements are unnecessary. You just need a few high-leverage principles.

The largest benefit to being lean is just how much time you'll have to focus on other aspects of your life. Long gone are the countless hours spent scouring fitness blogs and books, hoping to find that perfect formula to get shredded. Now you can spend that time with your kids, taking relaxing vacations with your spouse, or pursuing other passions.

For the first time in your life, "get back in shape" will no longer be a recurring item on the New Year's resolution list. That's an immensely liberating feeling.

I would love to hear your success stories from *Hack Your Fitness*. Please email me at jay@hackyour.fitness and share with me your experience hacking fitness.

Get ready to be the envy of all your friends. Get ready to be known as a "genetic freak." Get ready to celebrate your freedom. You are now part of an elite group that has learned how to hack fitness. Join us in the inner circle: http://hackyour.fitness/innercircle.

KEY TAKEAWAYS

- ◗ The most important rule over the next twelve weeks if your progress stalls is don't panic.
- ◗ If you're not progressing, make sure you're in 100 percent compliance with your diet and giving max effort on your workouts before changing anything.

- One common mistake during the twelve weeks is not recalculating your calorie budget as your weight goes down. Recalculate your TDEE every two weeks, and redo your calorie numbers based on that new figure.
- Weight loss can be slow if you're gaining new muscle. Focus on the visible changes your body is undergoing by taking weekly progress pictures.
- In the end, remember that we're about fat loss, not necessarily weight loss.
- Your body will cling to body fat as you approach single-digit body fat percentage, which makes it very challenging to break through and reach single digits.
- The more progress people make, the more they think they deserve to cheat on their diet. Avoid falling into this trap.
- Laziness during the final weeks is the biggest reason most people don't achieve single-digit body fat.
- If you're following *Hack Your Fitness* to the letter and are still stuck, you can implement strategic cardio after you fast on rest days to get you over the hump.
- A final strategy for dealing with stalled progress is The Regroup— one (and only one) big cheat meal where you go nuts and don't worry with tracking. This helps reset your mind and body for the final push.
- When the twelve weeks are over and maintenance starts, recalculate your TDEE based on your ending weight. Your daily calorie budget is now equal to your TDEE.
- You can add calories back to your weekly budget however you want, but two popular methods are replenishing your rest day budgets

(suggested route) or stockpiling calories for the weekend. It's up to you and your lifestyle.

- If you want to bulk up, first lean down to single-digit body fat before beginning your bulk.

- You can employ calculated cheating to enjoy festivities without stressing over your calories or macros.

- When going out to eat for a big occasion, get 90 percent of your lean protein in ahead of time.

- If your big meal falls on a rest day and you can't move your workouts, an advanced strategy you can use is a twenty-four-hour fast leading up to the big meal. You want to fast from dinner the night before to dinner that night.

- Regardless of what strategy you use, remember to have fun at your big event!

- You can use a light cardio session the morning after drinking to sober yourself up and avoid the temptation of indulging in unhealthy foods.

- If your lifestyle dictates that you can't skip breakfast, you'll have to shift your fasting window. As long as you fast for sixteen hours and feed for eight, you're good.

- When you travel, scope out your destination ahead of time to locate grocery stores and gyms.

- If you can't find a gym with a squat rack when you travel, stick to your rest day calories during your trip, and avoid cardio or dumbbell workouts as replacements for your regular workouts.

ACTION STEPS

- Be honest with yourself during these twelve weeks. Make sure you're 100 percent compliant on both the diet and exercise side of this program. At the end of the day, you only have yourself to answer to for your choices, and you are responsible for everything you put in your mouth.

- Use the strategies in this chapter if you're doing everything right and not seeing the progress you should. Try only one change at a time.

- Once the twelve weeks are over, recalculate your TDEE based on your ending weight, and add your calories back to your weekly budget for maintenance.

- Remember that the only way to enjoy this new life you've made for yourself is to view this program as the beginning of a lifestyle change, not a temporary fix.

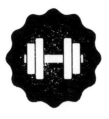

EPILOGUE

HACK THE HACK (THE TL;DR VERSION)

There is a small percentage of elite readers who are true world-class hackers that will have skimmed the table of contents and come directly to this section. These are the high achievers in the "just tell me what to do" crowd. If you've found yourself here without reading a single page of the book, I applaud your efficiency. This is for you.

INTRODUCTION

- This book is not a "get fit quick" scheme. Short of liposuction, overnight weight loss is not possible. Lasting results require patience.
- True fitness is more of a mental challenge than a physical one because you need the willpower to change your diet.
- Commit to making a lifestyle change that will radically improve your life.

PSYCHOLOGY

- Working out in the morning jump-starts your day and eliminates the excuses you might have for skipping your workout after your day job is finished.
- Take some time to find your trigger. Why do you really want to get fit?
- After you do that, go find a picture of your ideal body and cut and paste it somewhere you can see it every day for the next twelve weeks. This is your videotape.

FOUNDATION

- Fitness is 85 percent diet and 15 percent exercise—you can't out-work a bad diet.
- Proper nutrition is a way of eating for life, not a diet you pick up and put down.
- Regardless of our genetic predisposition, we have the power to move up and down the body-type scale if we so desire.
- Don't believe the lie that living with single-digit body fat is miserable. Contrary to popular belief, it's not all about bland foods and nonstop cardio.
- The saying, "Abs are made in the kitchen," is true, even if we don't like to admit it.
- You don't need cardio to get ripped.
- The Law of Energy Balance (Calories In vs. Calories Out), the Law of Macronutrient Balance, and the Law of Food Choices are the Three Laws of Nutrition you need to know to get ripped.
- Take an honest look at your diet, and start making changes today.
- Stop with the cardio. It's awful, and you don't have to do it anymore.

COUNTING CALORIES

- Counting calories is a necessary evil that separates those who are truly lean from those who look skinny but are technically fat (skinny fat).
- The Law of Energy Balance (Calories In vs. Calories Out) has the biggest impact on your nutrition.
- People struggle with calories in two ways: underestimating the number of calories they eat and thinking they need more calories than they actually do.
- Figuring out how many calories you burn every day comes from multiplying your basal metabolic rate by your daily activity factor.
- A pound of body fat is roughly equivalent to 3,500 calories, so in order to lose a pound a week, you need to operate at a caloric deficit of 3,500 calories for the week.
- If you slash your calories too aggressively, your body will go into starvation mode and do everything it can to hold on to that fat.
- Most people can expect to lose 1 to 1.5 pounds per week with *Hack Your Fitness*.
- Calculate your basal metabolic rate (using the formula or Google), then multiply that by 1.2 (the appropriate daily activity factor for most people) to determine your daily maintenance calories (TDEE).

INTERMITTENT FASTING

- Fasting for twenty-four hours or less will not slow down your metabolism.
- You don't have to eat six meals a day to get fit.
- Intermittent fasting (IF) is the most effective way to maintain a caloric deficit over a long period of time.

- IF is not a diet that dictates what you can eat, but rather a schedule for when you can eat.
- Your day is split into two windows with IF—fasting and feeding—with the fasting window being longer than the feeding window.
- Your body burns stored body fat in a fasted state, not your muscles.
- Some benefits of IF are that you see immediate results and your days of endless meal prep are over. Also, when you eat, you get to eat big.
- There are four IF protocols, and for the purposes of this program, I recommend 16:8.
- With 16:8, eating two or three meals during your feeding window is recommended compared to snacking because big meals are easier to track.
- You don't have to use IF to see results with Hack Your Fitness as long as you abide by the Laws of Nutrition, particularly the Law of Energy Balance.
- If you're going to use IF, start practicing it today.

TRACKING MACROS

- Every calorie is comprised of three macronutrients: protein, carbohydrates, and fat. Each macronutrient serves crucial functions within your body.
- If you know the macronutrient composition of a food item, you can use 4-4-9 to determine the number of calories it has.
- When you adhere to the Laws of Energy Balance and Macronutrient Balance, food choice is not that important.
- But you can't achieve long-term success with bad foods as a regular part of your diet.

- On workout days (three times a week), protein will constitute 45 percent of your daily caloric intake, and on rest days (four times a week), protein will be 55 percent of your calories.
- On workout days, your remaining calories will be 40 percent carbs and 15 percent fat. On rest days, it's more of an even split: 20 percent carbs and 25 percent fat.
- Don't listen to people who say carbs are bad or that you shouldn't eat fat. Those people are idiots. Your body needs the right combination of carbs and fat in conjunction with the proper protein intake.
- Ditch supplements, and chew your calories.
- Remember that weight loss is not linear. The amount of weight you start out losing the first few weeks won't be the amount you lose every week.
- Body fat calipers are the most affordable and easiest way to measure body fat.
- Using your daily calorie budget, determine the amount of each macronutrient you need to consume on workout and rest days. Keep in mind that your calorie budget is roughly 40 percent lower on rest days compared to workout days.
- Go to http://hackyour.fitness/resources to download the free Macro Calculator.
- Then go to MyFitnessPal.com and download the app.
- Buy a pair of body fat calipers and a food scale.
- Establish your routine—tracking, weighing, and measuring body fat—and begin practicing it to ingrain this behavior as a new habit in your life.

ALCOHOL

- For the twelve weeks you're on Hack Your Fitness, you can't drink.

- The bad news is that booze blocks fat oxygenation and hijacks your metabolism, meaning everything you eat after you drink gets stored as fat.

- Alcohol lowers your testosterone, which is needed for building muscles.

- But don't worry, you will get to drink again after the initial twelve weeks. When that time comes, limit yourself to drinking once a week.

- Bid farewell to drinking for the next twelve weeks. (Yes, I really mean it.)

COMPOUND LIFTS

- The principle of progressive overload says that in order to get stronger over time, you must increase the number of reps or amount of weight you're lifting each time you work out.

- Every strength-training program should include the three main compound lifts: squat, deadlift, and overhead press.

- You can keep your gym membership if you want, but you don't need it for Hack Your Fitness. All you need is a squat rack with barbell and bench setup.

- Compound lifts have the highest EPOC, or afterburn effect, of any exercise. Your body is still recovering up to forty-eight hours after a lift.

- The single most important thing you can do while working out is track your lifts.

- You need two days of rest between the squat and deadlift.

- Squatting on Sundays gets your most physically demanding lift out of the way before your week even starts.
- Hack Your Fitness uses reverse pyramid training, or starting with your heaviest set and working down from there.
- The rep range will be between six and eight reps because you're lifting heavy.
- On rest days, you truly need to rest. Your body needs time to recover.
- Besides the squat rack and bench setup, all you need for working out are shoes with a noncompressible heel (such as Converse All-Stars) and a workout log.
- Find a gym that has a squat rack and bench setup, or buy that equipment (plus the barbell) for your house if you have room to spare. Buy yourself some inexpensive workout shoes, and decide how you want to track your lifts.
- Commit to working out on Sundays. You'll be thankful you did come Monday morning.

SQUAT

- Regardless of your fitness goals, the squat is the most important exercise you can do.
- When you go to squat, set the rack so the bar height is even with the middle of your chest.
- Step backward out of the rack to perform your squat, never forward.
- Your bar path as you squat should be a straight line.
- Get your ass in the hole when you squat by dropping your hips below the level of the top of your knees.
- For all the compound lifts: Breathe in at the top of your movement,

hold your breath during the movement, and breathe out on your way back to the starting position. This is known as the Valsalva maneuver.

○ Point your feet out thirty degrees and make sure your knees follow that angle instead of coming together when you squat.

○ When you squat, focus on a point ten to fifteen feet in front of you instead of looking at the mirror or up at the ceiling.

○ While resting between sets, visualize your form for the next set.

PRESS

○ The overhead press (or simply the press) works your triceps, shoulders, and upper chest, making it a more useful lift than other upper-body workouts like bicep curls or the bench press.

○ Bar height setup should be mid-chest, your grip should be slightly wider than your shoulders, and you must keep your forearms straight. (No chicken wings!)

○ Save your wrists by gripping the bar in the base of your palm.

○ Your feet should be shoulder-width apart.

○ The angle of your feet doesn't really matter like it does with the squat.

○ When you're ready, unrack the bar, take a deep breath, and push the bar straight up.

○ Don't bend your knees for an extra bounce.

DEADLIFT

○ The deadlift movement is simple: pull the bar with straight arms up the path of your legs until you're standing upright.

- Although the movement is easy to learn, don't be a hero and add too much weight too quickly. That's a recipe for injury.

- For your stance: Keep your feet eight to twelve inches apart, toes pointing out thirty degrees, with the middle of the bar centered between your feet.

- When the bar comes up, it should be as close to your shins as possible without risking injury. If you look at your foot from heel to toes, draw a horizontal line in the middle, and that should be your starting bar position.

- The width of your grip should be just outside your legs.

- When you bend down to grab the bar, keep your back straight. Curving your spine during the deadlift could cause serious injury.

- The ideal hip depth for the deadlift is about half the depth of a squat, and your knees should shove out when you reach down for the bar.

- As always, don't forget to use the Valsalva maneuver during this lift.

- At the top of your movement, when you're standing up straight, don't hyperextend your back, thrust your hips forward, or shrug your shoulders.

- This is not an arm exercise—use your back and hips to pull the bar up. Your arms are simply clamps to hold the bar.

- When you come down from the lockout (upright) position, the bar must come to a dead stop at the bottom of your movement. (Hence, the deadlift!)

- Don't bounce at the bottom of your movement!

PLATEAUS

- If you're not progressing, make sure you're in 100 percent compliance with your diet and giving max effort on your workouts before changing anything.

○ One common mistake during the twelve weeks is not recalculating your calorie budget as your weight goes down. Recalculate your TDEE every two weeks, and redo your calorie numbers based on that new figure.

○ Weight loss can be slow if you're gaining new muscle. Focus on the visible changes your body is undergoing by taking weekly progress pictures.

○ In the end, remember that we're about fat loss, not necessarily weight loss.

○ Your body will cling to body fat as you approach single-digit body fat percentage, which makes it very challenging to break through and reach single digits.

○ The more progress people make, the more they think they deserve to cheat on their diet. Avoid falling into this trap.

○ Laziness during the final weeks is the biggest reason most people don't achieve single-digit body fat.

○ If you're following Hack Your Fitness to the letter and are still stuck, you can implement strategic cardio after you fast on rest days to get you over the hump.

○ A final strategy for dealing with stalled progress is The Regroup—one (and only one) big cheat meal where you go nuts and don't worry with tracking. This helps reset your mind and body for the final push.

○ When the twelve weeks are over and maintenance starts, recalculate your TDEE based on your ending weight. Your daily calorie budget is now equal to your TDEE.

○ If you want to bulk up, lean down to single-digit body fat before beginning your bulk.

LIFESTYLE AND TRAVEL

- You can employ calculated cheating to enjoy festivities without stressing over your calories or macros.
- When going out to eat for a big occasion, get 90 percent of your lean protein in ahead of time.
- If your big meal falls on a rest day and you can't move your workouts, an advanced strategy you can use is a twenty-four-hour fast leading up to the big meal. You want to fast from dinner the night before to dinner that night.
- You can use a light cardio session the morning after drinking to sober yourself up and avoid the temptation of indulging in unhealthy foods.
- When you travel, scope out your destination ahead of time to locate grocery stores and gyms.
- If you can't find a gym with a squat rack when you travel, stick to your rest day calories during your trip, and avoid cardio or dumbbell workouts as replacements for your regular workouts.

CONCLUSION

- Be honest with yourself during these twelve weeks. Make sure you're 100 percent compliant on both the diet and exercise side of this program. At the end of the day, you only have yourself to answer to for your choices, and you are responsible for everything you put in your mouth.
- Remember that the only way to enjoy this new life you've made for yourself is to view this program as the beginning of a lifestyle change, not a temporary fix.

Good Protein	Good Carbs (Fibrous)	Good Fats
Chicken Breast (no skin)	Asparagus	Almonds, Almond Butter
Chicken Tenderloin	Broccoli	Brazil Nuts
Clams	Brussel Sprouts	Canola oil
Cod	Cabbage	Cashews, Cashew Butter
Crab	Carrots	Fish Fat/Oil
Egg Whites	Cauliflower	Flaxseed/Oil
Flank Steak	Celery	Hazelnuts
Halibut	Cucumbers	Natural peanut butter
Lean Ground Beef	Eggplant	Nuts & seeds
Lean Ground Turkey	Green Beans	Olive oil
Lobster	Green/Red Peppers	Pecans
Low Fat Cottage Cheese	Kale	Pistachios
Low Fat Greek Yogurt	Lettuce	Pumpkin Seed/Oil
Mackerel	Mushrooms	Sunflower Seeds
Mussels	Onions	Walnuts
Octopus	Radish	
Orange Roughy	Snow Peas	
Oysters	Spinach	
Pork Tenderloin	Squash	
Protein Powder	Tomatoes	
Salmon	Zucchini	
Scallops		
Seabass	**Good Carbs (Starchy)**	
Shrimp	Barley	
Sirloin Steak	Beans	
Snapper	Brown Rice	
Swordfish	· Buckwheat	
Tilapia	Chickpeas	
Top/Bottom Round Steak	Corn	
Tuna Fish	Cream of Rice	
Turkey Breast (no skin)	Lentils	
	Oat Bran	
	Oatmeal	
	Potatoes	
	Pumpernickel	
	Quinoa	
	Rye	
	Sourdough	
	Sweet Potatoes	
	Whole Wheat	
	Whole Wheat Tortilla	
	Yams	

OK Carbs (Moderation)
Dairy Products
Fruit Juices
Fruits (All)
Tortillas
Whole Wheat Bread
Whole Wheat Pasta

Bad Protein (Avoid!)	Bad Carbs (Avoid!)	Bad Fats (Avoid!)
Bacon	Brown Sugar	Saturated Animal Fats
Ground Beef	Biscuits	High Fat Dairy (cheese)
Processed/Deli Meats	Candy	Lunchmeat
Sausage	Chocolates	Margarine
Steak (most cuts)	Donuts	Non Dairy Creamer
	Fried Foods	Palm Oil
	Frosting	Poultry Skin
	Fruit drinks	Shortening
	Honey	Transfat from Baked Goods
	Ice Cream	Transfat from Deep Frying
	Molasses	
	Pastries	
	Pies	
	Potato Chips	
	Soda	
	Sweet Rolls	
	White bread	
	White Rice	
	White sugar	

APPENDIX

THE HACK YOUR DIET GUIDE

(Opposite page)

THE ALTERNATE EXERCISE GUIDE
FRONT SQUAT

To the casual gym bro, the front squat may seem like an advanced and almost daunting exercise. Other than Crossfitters or Olympic weightlifters, you rarely see anyone doing them. While it is a movement that requires a certain level of education, I'm here to tell you that it is actually not that technical or difficult to master. It also happens to be one of the best barbell squat variations out there, which is why it has earned its spot in the elite *Hack Your Fitness* training program.

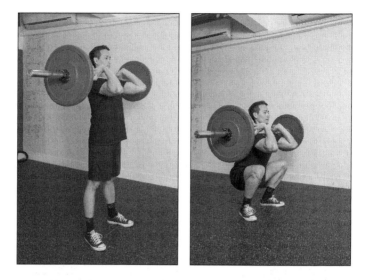

The front squat is not as wholesome of a movement as the back squat due to the simple fact that it does not involve the entire posterior chain. The other big difference between the back squat and the front squat is that there is no hip drive in the front squat. The lifter's hips are directly under the bar during this movement, so the focus is less on the hamstrings and more on the glutes. If you think your ass is sore the day after back squatting, front squatting takes this to a whole new level.

During the front squat, the back must be kept in a very upright and vertical position to ensure a vertical line bar path. This requires the lifter to open up his hips when performing the movement and ensures that the knees move forward on the same path/angle that the feet are positioned.

You want to keep your chest up and back upright, similar to your upper-body position during the press.

The bar setup should be the exact same as the back squat, with the bar racked at the mid-chest level. You won't be able to front squat as much as you back squat, but it still is a great assistance exercise, which I recommend only after pushing yourself in the back squat to failure. Your stance will be the same as the back squat, with feet slightly wider than shoulder-length apart and toes pointed out at thirty degrees.

The front squat is an awkward movement if you are just starting off. The hardest thing to master is the bar position on the shoulders. Many people make the mistake of putting the bar too high and choking themselves in the neck, or placing the bar too low only for it to fall off midexercise. Bar placement is of paramount importance, which is why it can be awkward at first and many people shy away from it.

The most important thing to remember is not to have the bar too close to your neck, as this can get very dangerous under a load if you happen to get in a pinch. Always err on the side of caution and rack the bar or drop it if something doesn't feel right.

The bar should rest on the meat of your deltoids. For novices who do not have developed shoulders yet, this may be resting on the bone, which could cause some discomfort at first. All the more reason to keep training your presses!

Wrist flexibility is often another issue when it comes to front squatting. As with the press, there should be no load pressure on your wrists whatsoever once the bar is in place and your elbows are up. If there is, you can try releasing one or two of your fingers (pinkie, ring) for comfort. At the minimum you need your thumb, index, and middle fingers for grip. The width of your grip will be directly affected by the flexibility of your wrists. Feel free to take a wider grip if necessary.

Another option is taking a position with your arms crossed. This is called the California front squat, and I personally find this positioning to be less stable as you add load, and difficult to rack at the end of a set. The important thing to remember is that whichever arm position you choose, make sure you keep your elbows up and locked at a ninety-degree angle to your body to ensure upright form.

You'll find as you get fatigued in the set that your first instinct will be to drop your elbows from the ninety-degree angle. Once this happens, your set is all but finished. Resist the urge, and focus on keeping elbows up, chest out, and back straight.

Five steps to proper front squatting:

1. Body upright (Remember the vertical bar path.)
2. Chest up
3. Elbows up
4. Hips open
5. Knees out (Follow the same path as your feet.)

CALF RAISES

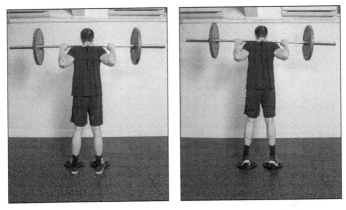

The calf raise is another good accessory exercise you'll want to do if you have under developed calf muscles, or "chicken legs." If you're like me and resisted leg day for most of your fitness career, calf training is something you'll definitely want to implement regularly. Most gyms have both sitting and standing calf raise machines. This is the only exception in *Hack Your Fitness* where I will actually recommend you use one of those machines versus using the rack. The machines were well designed for comfort and isolate the range of motion necessary to target the calf, so if you see one of these machines available and it's the end of your workout, feel free to jump on it.

That said, as hackers, we know that we can actually do this exercise in a squat rack with a barbell. To do so is actually quite simple. Rack the bar as if you were doing a back squat, only with the resting pins racked one notch higher than normal. Then put a couple of plates down on the floor (I use twenty-four pounds) as a makeshift plank to step up onto for the calf raise. Since the plates on the floor provide elevation, you see why we want to rack the barbell one notch higher, so that it rests nicely on your traps when you begin the exercise.

Step up into the rack, and use the floor plates to leverage your movement in the rack. I like to lean in and use the front of the rack as a support surface to slide the barbell up and down as opposed to free standing with the bar to do the raises. I find this helpful when adding load. I'll be completely honest with you: doing calf raises in a squat rack is not pretty, but if you need a hack, there you go. If done properly, it works.

BENCH PRESS

The bench press is the single most recognized weight-lifting exercise in the world. It is nearly synonymous with

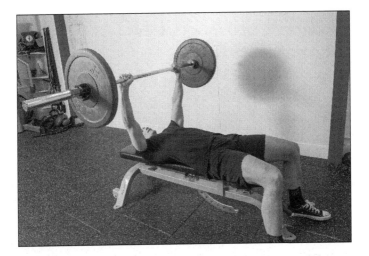

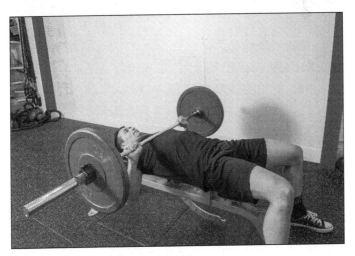

weight training, as evidenced by the fact that a person's entire fitness tends be gauged by a single number that answers the question, "How much do you bench, bro?" The bench press and bicep curl are usually the first two exercises fitness newbies try because, naturally, all guys want to have a big chest and bulging biceps. Even people who never work out regularly have probably at some point attempted the bench press. It's just one of those things that all guys like to do.

The bench press is arguably the most effective way to develop pure upper strength (compared to the press, which works your entire body), and that is due to the simple fact that you can load more weight on the bench press with a spotter than you can on the press. The more you load, the more you grow.

While benching may be the most common exercise in the gym, it's also one of the most dangerous ones, especially as you push yourself to failure. I myself am embarrassed to say that I've tried to max out without a spotter, failed, and had to scream for help from the gym-bro meatheads to save my neck. Word of caution: If you are benching to failure, *always* use a spotter.

Let's begin. Your starting position should be such that when you lie down, your chest should be positioned well in front of the bar. What this means is that your body should be positioned far enough down toward the foot of the bench so that when you reach up to grab the bar, your arms are not perpendicular, but rather slightly reaching up behind you.

As you lie down and gaze straight up at the ceiling, you should be looking at the front side of the bar (the side closest to your feet). Take a grip similar to the press where the weight of the bar rests on the heels of the palm so as not to pressure your wrists during the movement. Always wrap your thumbs around the bar in a closed grip. Never use a thumbless grip.

Lift the bar up out of the safety pins and into the starting position. Your arms should be perpendicular now at a ninety-degree angle to your body. Take a deep breath, and bring the bar down to your chest so it hits midsternum (nipple line). As soon as the bar touches your chest, drive the bar back up to the starting position. Remember: If the bar doesn't touch your chest, it doesn't count as a full rep.

Don't bounce at the bottom of the rep, don't arch your back, and don't lift your feet off the floor. You sometimes see bros in the gym benching with their feet up as if they are trying to do crunches at the same time, claiming it "isolates the core." That's just idiotic. Keep your feet firmly planted on the ground, and use them to drive your movement.

There are literally thousands of pages worth of literature that you can find on benching technique, but ultimately my old saying. "Don't think; just do," comes into play here. Don't overthink the mechanics of the bench press too much.

The quickest way to learn is to get under the bar, start with low weight, learn the movement, keep practicing, and iterate.

There are many variations of the bench press that can easily be manipulated by widening or narrowing the grip. The narrower the grip, the more you'll work your inner chest and triceps. The wider the grip, the more outer chest you'll use. For maximum effectiveness, choose the closest grip to shoulder width that you can manage.

INCLINE PRESS

This is a pure assistance exercise, which is why it is the last of the three presses you will perform on push day. By the time you get to this exercise, you will be pretty well fatigued and most of your work (if you have been pushing at max effort to failure) will already be completed with the press and the bench press.

The incline bench works more of the upper chest and shoulder muscles than the flat bench does and is a great exercise to complete your barbell push circuit. The reason it's included is because most people get fatigued very quickly when performing the overhead press, and their muscles give out long before they can appropriately overload and stress them. Progressive overload requires either additional weight or additional volume, and many

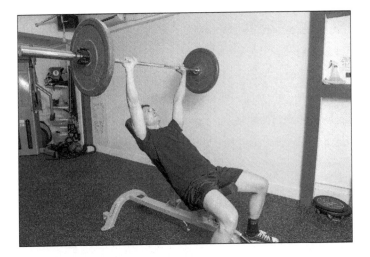

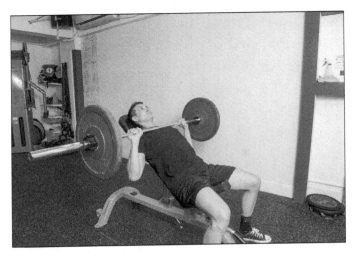

lifters (myself included) end up being "stuck" at the same overhead press weight for weeks at a time with extremely slow progress. Adding in two sets of incline press will ensure you properly overload your upper body so you can make incremental strength gains for your next push day.

The movement is the same as the flat bench press with just two points to remember:

1. The bar path should be vertical as always.

2. Make sure your ass stays on the incline bench. Don't get into the bad habit of arching your back or raising your ass in the air to assist with your movement.

BARBELL ROW

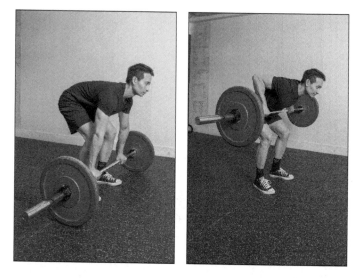

The barbell row is the best rowing exercise available. Don't waste time with that pulldown machine or the cable row machine when you can do your rows from the comfort of your own squat rack.

The key to this, just like the deadlift, is that the movement begins with the bar on the floor, and then ends with the bar on the floor for each and every rep (like the deadlift). No bouncing. Approach the bar as you would a deadlift with the feet positioned the same. Take a double overhand grip slightly wider than shoulder-length apart, and make sure that when bent over, your lower back is not rounded but held in extension, similar to the start of a deadlift.

Keep your chest up, take a deep breath in, and pull the bar off the floor up to the area near your lower rib cage. Then return the bar to the floor and exhale. That's one rep. Don't try to hold the bar at the top of the movement. Make sure your eyes are fixated to a point a few feet in front of you and not straight ahead in the mirror because you think you look badass.

SHRUGS

Barbell shrugs are often overlooked by many gym bros, but they do much more for you than just giving you those nice flared traps that Tom Hardy had in the movie *Warrior*. Traps, in addition to being a staple of all bodybuilding meatheads out there, are actually functional in that they will help build out the muscles that you will need to support the bar in a back squat. Traps also assist with overall shoulder strength and function.

Shrugs should be performed heavy, and the movement

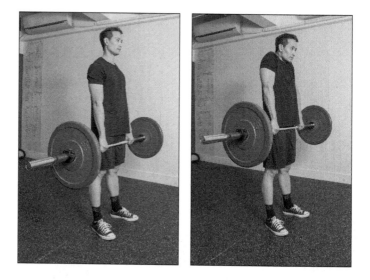

is a quick shrug up and back down to the racked position. There is no need to do a slow deliberate shrug or to hold the shrug position at the top like you see some folks doing in the gym. The movement is explosive and heavy. Make sure to keep your chest up and body upright as you perform the movement, and each rep should be done individually like a deadlift: up, down, and then bar back to the racked position.

THE DYNAMIC DUO: DIPS AND CHIN-UPS

Both dips and chin-ups are great exercises that work a variety of muscle groups, which make them ideal for *Hack Your Fitness*. They are hands down the two best nonbarbell exercises out there and the only two that I recommend for our program that can't be done with a barbell and rack.

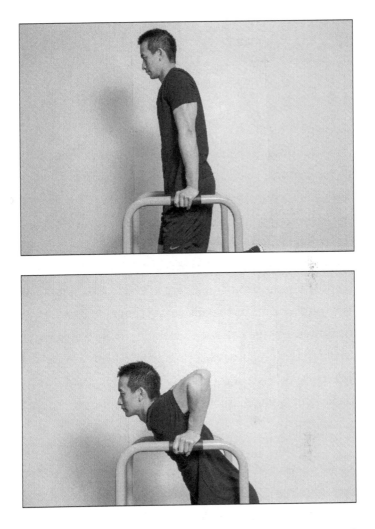

(Mind you, my rack at home has a chin-up bar up top and a separate dipping attachment.) As you get stronger and move beyond bodyweight repetitions, you will want to pick up a dipping belt similar to this so you can add load.

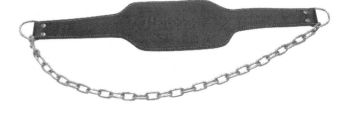

One Harbinger dipping belt will set you back around thirty dollars but will last you a lifetime. If you lift heavy for the next thirty years, that's just a dollar a year. Mine is going twelve years strong, and it still looks brand spanking new.

Once you get stronger and start using the weighted dipping belt for dips and chin-ups, remember to calculate your "working weight" as the entire weight being used—your body weight plus the added weight plates. Since we're working with reverse pyramid training, our second set will be 90 percent of the total weight. It may require you to do some quick math, but this is the proper way to load these lifts.

As an example, if I weigh 155 pounds and am able to perform six chin-ups with a forty-five-pound plate (for a total of 200 pounds), then my second set would be 180 pounds (200 pounds × 90 percent), so I would switch the forty-five-pound plate for a twenty-five-pound plate.

Dips are a great exercise that works the shoulders, lower pecs, and triceps. I've even heard the dip being referred to as the "squat of the upper body." The ability to add load to them via a dipping belt makes them much more useful than the push-up.

Make sure you use a proper dipping attachment to your squat rack or use parallel bars. Don't be an idiot and try to dip between two folding chairs. That's the quickest way to injury. The complete movement of the dip is all the way down (until the chest is deep and the top of your triceps are perpendicular to the bars) and then all the way up (until arms are straight and your body is fully upright).

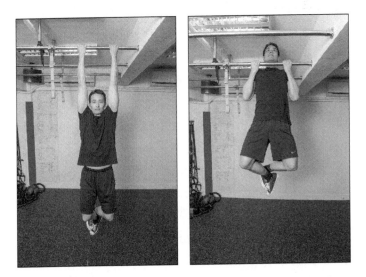

Chin-ups are pretty self-explanatory. The one important note to make is that the proper movement is all the way up (chin above the bar) and *all the way down*. Most people try to "cheat" and not go down all the way. Doing this would be the half squat equivalent of a chin-up. Make sure each rep counts, and go all the way down.

Lastly, don't you dare think about "kipping." If you don't know what kipping is, Google it.

BAR PLACEMENT FOR SQUATS: HIGH OR LOW?

There are two variations of bar placement when performing the squat: high bar or low bar. You usually see most people using the conventional high bar placement when they squat. The bar rests mostly on the lifter's traps, and the squat range of motion and back angle is more upright. I squatted with a high bar for many years until I recently discovered the low bar placement.

Without going into all the technical differences between the two, the honest truth is that it doesn't really matter. Some like to argue that you can lift more weight in the low bar position, which is what intrigued me to begin with and prompted me to switch. In the end, just pick what feels right for you. Low bar squatting takes a bit of adjustment, but I've found that, because of the forward back angle, I tend to look at the mirror in front of me less (which is a good thing) and focus more on the range of motion through muscle memory.

Can I squat more weight? Not really. My squat is pretty weak since I started squatting so late in my fitness career, so I never really got to enjoy that benefit. Low bar squatting often feels awkward for newbies, and it takes some time to adjust and learn how to position the bar so as not to add pressure to your wrists.

In the end, the only reason you would actually *need* to squat low bar is if you are a powerlifter because powerlifting is all about the amount of weight you can put up.

When performing the low bar squat, the barbell should be positioned just under the spine of the scapula (the bump you feel on your shoulder blade). When done properly this will create a "shelf" that will allow the bar to be locked into place by your grip.

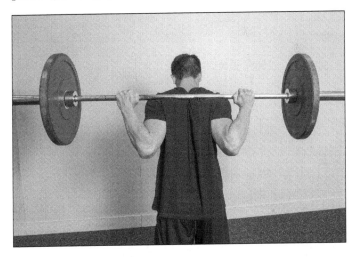

The correct grip keeps the hands above the bar at all times and the weight of the bar on the back. Your hands and wrists should never be supporting any weight. They are simply there to lock the bar in place. You should experience some slight discomfort in this position initially as it is not a "natural" feel per se.

Depending on your flexibility, you will want your wrists positioned as closely together as possible. Wider grips are dangerous when squatting because they don't provide the "lock" that you need to keep the bar in place, especially as you go up in weight.

EXERCISE SUBSTITUTION MATRIX

Day 1: Squat	Alternative 1	Alternative 2 (travel only)
Back Squat	n/a	Seated Leg Press/Hack Squat
Front Squat	Bulgarian Split Squat	Leg Extension/Leg Curls
Calf Raise	Seated/Leg Press Calf Raise	Dumbbell Calf Raise

Day 2: Push	Alternative 1	Alternative 2 (travel only)
Overhead press	n/a	Standing Dumbbell OH Press
Bench Press	Flat Bench Dumbbell Press	Seated Machine Chest Press
Incline Press	Incline Bench Dumbbell Press	Pec-Dec Machine
Dips	Dumbbell Pull-Over	Dumbbell Fly/Cable Fly

Day 3: Pull	Alternative 1	Alternative 2 (travel only)
Deadlift	n/a	One-Arm Dumbbell Deadlift
Chin Ups	Lateral Pull Down	Close-Grip Pull Down
Bent Over Row	Bent Over Dumbbell Row	Seated Cable Row
Shrugs	Dumbbell Shrugs	Dumbbell Lateral Raise

NOTES

- I shouldn't have even included this, because there is basically no reason you won't be able to do all the lifts I prescribe in *Hack Your Fitness* if you have access to a squat rack.
- Use alternate exercises very sparingly. Remember, barbell compound lifts are king.
- Free weights (barbells/dumbbells) are always preferred over machines. Use machines only if you have to.
- I deliberated long and hard on including the Alternate Exercise 2 column, but I realize that shit happens. Don't be an idiot. Use these extremely sparingly, only if you have a gun to your head, and never more than one week continuously when on travel. The sooner you can get back to barbell compound lifts, the better.

THE HACK YOUR FITNESS TWELVE-WEEK WORKOUT LOG

(See next page)

MYFITNESSPAL SETUP INSTRUCTIONS

MyFitnessPal by Under Armour is hands down the best calorie counter and macro tracker I've tested, and scores of my coaching clients also swear by it. Not only does it have the world's largest nutrition and calorie database comprising of over five million foods; it also has a convenient barcode-scanning function by which you can scan foods and load the data directly into your tracker. Last but not least, it's free.

		Reps Range	Day 1: Squat Back Squat 6-8	Front Squat 6-8	Calf Raise 10-12	Reps Range	Day 2: Push OH Press 6-8	Bench Press 6-8	Incline Press 6-8	Dips 6-8	Reps Range	Day 3: Pull Deadlift 6-8	Chin Ups 6-8	Barbell Row 6-8	Shrugs 10-12
Date	Body Weight														
Week 1	___	Set 1				Set 1					Set 1				
		Set 2				Set 2					Set 2				
Week 2	___	Set 1				Set 1					Set 1				
		Set 2				Set 2					Set 2				
Week 3	___	Set 1				Set 1					Set 1				
		Set 2				Set 2					Set 2				
Week 4	___	Set 1				Set 1					Set 1				
		Set 2				Set 2					Set 2				
Week 5	___	Set 1				Set 1					Set 1				
		Set 2				Set 2					Set 2				
Week 6	___	Set 1				Set 1					Set 1				
		Set 2				Set 2					Set 2				
Week 7	___	Set 1				Set 1					Set 1				
		Set 2				Set 2					Set 2				
Week 8	___	Set 1				Set 1					Set 1				
		Set 2				Set 2					Set 2				
Week 9	___	Set 1				Set 1					Set 1				
		Set 2				Set 2					Set 2				
Week 10	___	Set 1				Set 1					Set 1				
		Set 2				Set 2					Set 2				
Week 11	___	Set 1				Set 1					Set 1				
		Set 2				Set 2					Set 2				
Week 12	___	Set 1				Set 1					Set 1				
		Set 2				Set 2					Set 2				

Here are the exact steps you need to take to download MyFitnessPal and set it up on your phone to start tracking your data today.

PART I: DOWNLOAD AND REGISTER

Go to the Google Play Store or iTunes App Store and search for MyFitnessPal. Click on the blue icon that says *Calorie Counter – MyFitnessPal* and select *Install*. (Instructions will be similar for iPhone users. Get the initial setup done, and skip down to Part II.)

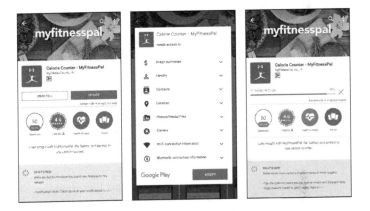

Click the green *Accept* button to continue. This should take about a minute or so (size is 19.55 MB) to download and install. Click the green *Open* button to launch the application and begin the setup process.

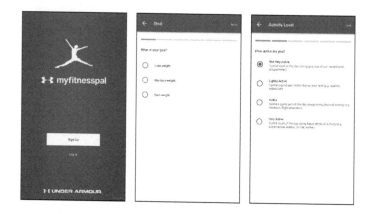

At the home screen select *Sign Up*. You have the option to sign up with email or Facebook. Choose whichever you like.

The next few screens are just initial setup screens. Note: Your answers here don't actually matter because all we care about is the tracking function for the app.

Next it will ask you "What is your goal?" and "How active are you?" Select *Not Very Active*.

Enter the following information on the following screens:

1. Gender, birthdate, and location
2. Height and current weight
3. Your goal weight (It doesn't matter what you put here.)
4. Underneath that, enter "Lose 2 lbs. per week" (but it doesn't actually matter)
5. Your email address, password, and username credentials

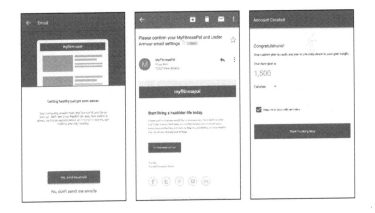

Select *No, don't send me emails.* Then you should receive an email at the registered email address asking you to "Confirm email settings." Click the blue button.

This will take you to a "Congratulations!" screen. Don't worry about the daily goal they say you should hit. We will go in and reconfigure everything. Click on the blue *Start Tracking Now* button.

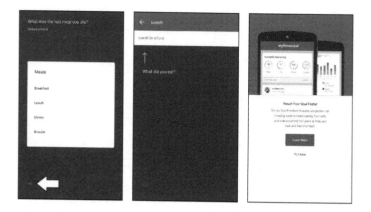

The screen will now say, "What was the last meal you ate?" Select anything or select *Skip* at the bottom left of the screen. You will come to a "Learn More" screen. Select *Not Now*.

PART II: SETTING YOUR GOALS

Finally, you are in the main screen. Go to the top left corner and select the menu button.

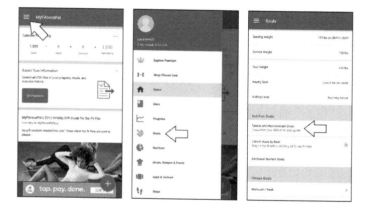

Select Goals and scroll down under the middle section
Nutrition Goals and select Calorie and Macronutrient
Goals.

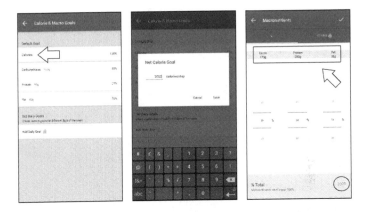

Under Default Goal, tap on Calories and input your calorie
budget for the day. Remember, it's higher if it's a training
day and lower if it's a rest day. (Yes, you must change this
every day for the free version.) Click Save.

Now set up your macronutrient ratios. Tap on any of the
macronutrients to enter your percentage.

If it's a training day: Carbs 40%; Protein 45%; Fat 15%

If it's a rest day: Carbs 20%; Protein 55%; Fat 25%

Check the bottom right hand of the screen. The number
should be a green 100%.

Tip: Take note of the grams of your macronutrients at the top of this screen. These are the daily gram amounts per macronutrient you need to hit. These numbers should be the same that you get from the Macro Calculator that is available as a free download at http://hackyour.fitness/resources. You'll be able to memorize these numbers for your training day and rest day after a while.

Click the check mark at the top right of the screen if everything looks right. Now your default goal is set.

PART III: TRACKING YOUR MACROS

Go back two screens to the main screen.

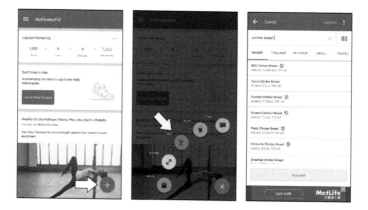

Click the + sign at the bottom right hand side of the screen. Click Food (the middle red button). Click on Lunch and start entering your food in the search bar at the top. (I use Tyson Chick Breast as an example here.)

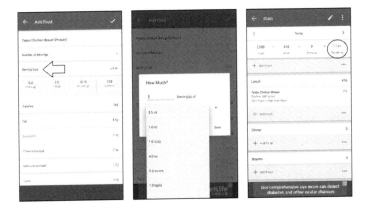

Tap on the Serving Size to manipulate based on food weight. In this example, I use 250g of chicken breast. As you add foods that you eat, MyFitnessPal will automatically deduct the calories from your daily budget at the top.

To check how your macronutrients add up over the course of the day, scroll to the bottom and select Nutrition.

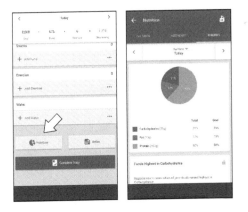

This screen shows you how many grams of each macronutrient you've eaten so far.

Warning: Do not be alarmed by the pie graph showing your macro percentage. This is simple a percentage based on what you've eaten so far in the day. Remember our macro goals from the earlier screen were Carb 200g, Protein 225g, and Fat 33g.

Now the fun begins. Complete the macro puzzle each day and try to hit your numbers as close as possible.

Once you find a few meals that you like to eat consistently, go to Menu and select Meals, Recipes & Foods.

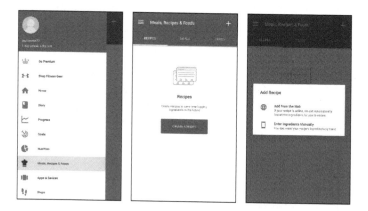

Click Create a Recipe. If the recipe is online, then select the first option. If not, select Enter Ingredients Manually. Enter a title for your meal and start adding ingredients.

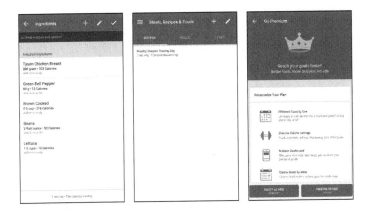

You might have to do some quick Google searching and conversions to get the right measurement units. Once you are done, click the check mark at the top right and select Save.

Now this recipe will be stored in your Meals, Recipes & Foods menu forever. Every time you have the same meal again, it's one click away to add it to your daily macros.

REMINDER: You must change your calorie goal each day based on if it's a training day or a rest day. Unfortunately, this is required of the free version. If you can't be bothered to change it every day, you can always pay for the premium version and Add Daily Goals in the Calorie & Macro Goals screen.

(At $10 per month, I'd rather just re-enter my goals every day. I feel it also keeps me aware on a daily basis what I need to aim for.)

Try to get as close as possible to your calorie and macronutrient goal each day.

This process may seem tedious at first, but after a day or two you will become proficient at using the app and it will take you less than a minute to log your macros in. Try to have fun with it.

That's it!

BIBLIOGRAPHY

BOOKS, WEBSITES, PRODUCTS, AND ARTICLES FOR FURTHER READING

BOOKS

Covey, Stephen R. *The 7 Habits of Highly Effective People: Powerful Lessons in Personal Change*. New York: Simon & Schuster, 2013.

Duhigg, Charles. *The Power of Habit: Why We Do What We Do in Life and Business*. New York: Random House, 2012.

Elrod, Hal. *The Miracle Morning: The Not-So-Obvious Secret Guaranteed to Transform Your Life before 8AM*. 2012.

Ferriss, Timothy. *The 4-Hour Body: An Uncommon Guide to Rapid Fat-Loss, Incredible Sex, and Becoming Superhuman*. New York: Crown Archetype, 2010.

Gawande, Atul. *The Checklist Manifesto: How to Get Things Right.* New York: Picador, 2010.

Greene, Robert. *Mastery.* New York: Penguin Books, 2013.

Holiday, Ryan. *The Obstacle Is the Way: The Little Book for Flipping Adversity into Opportunity.* Penguin Group USA, 2014.

Matthews, Michael. *Bigger Leaner Stronger: The Simple Science of Building the Ultimate Male Body.* Des Moines, IA: Waterbury, 2014.

Pilon, Brad. *Eat. Stop. Eat.* 2007.

Ries, Eric. *The Lean Startup: How Today's Entrepreneurs Use Continuous Innovation to Create Radically Successful Businesses.* New York: Crown Business, 2011.

Rippetoe, Mark. *Starting Strength: Basic Barbell Training.* Wichita Falls, TX: Aasgaard, 2011.

Schwartz, David Joseph. *The Magic of Thinking Big.* New York: Simon & Schuster, 1987.

Schwarzenegger, Arnold, and Bill Dobbins. *The New Encyclopedia of Modern Bodybuilding.* New York: Simon & Schuster, 1998.

Scott, S. J. *Habit Stacking: 97 Small Life Changes That Take Five Minutes or Less.* Printed by CreateSpace Independent Publishing Platform, 2014.

Sivers, Derek. *Anything You Want: 40 Lessons for a New Kind of Entrepreneur.* New York: Portfolio Penguin, 2015.

Strossen, Randall J. *Super Squats: How to Gain 30 Pounds of Muscle in 6 Weeks.* Nevada City, CA: IronMind Enterprises, 1989.

Venuto, Tom. *Burn the Fat, Feed the Muscle: Transform Your Body Forever Using the Secrets of the Leanest People in the World.* New York: Harmony, 2013.

Wansink, Brian. *Mindless Eating: Why We Eat More Than We Think.* New York: Bantam Books, 2007.

Willoughby, David P. *The Super-Athletes.* South Brunswick, NJ: A. S. Barnes, 1970.

WEBSITES

Berkhan, Martin. Leangains. http://www.leangains.com/.

Calorie King. http://www.calorieking.com/.

Fat Secret. http://www.fatsecret.com/.

Matthews, Michael. Legion Athletics. https://legionathletics.com/.

Matthews, Michael. Muscle for Life. http://www.muscleforlife.com/.

My Fitness Pal. https://www.myfitnesspal.com/.

Venuto, Tom. Burn the Fat Blog. http://www.burnthefatblog.com/.

PRODUCTS

AccuFitness. Accu-Measure Fitness 3000 Body Fat Caliper. http://www.accumeasurefitness.com/accu-measure-fitness-3000-body-fat-caliper.html.

Joseph Joseph. TriScale™. https://www.josephjoseph.com/en-rw/triscale.

ARTICLES

"Ask Men's Fitness: At What Age Does a Person's Metabolism Start to Significantly Slow?" *Men's Fitness*, September 24, 2014. http://www.mensfitness.com/weight-loss/burn-fat-fast/ask-mens-fitness-what-age-does-persons-metabolism-start-significantly-slow.

Bellisle, France, Regina Mcdevitt, and Andrew M. Prentice. "Meal Frequency and Energy Balance." *British Journal of Nutrition* 77, no. S1 (April 1997). doi: 10.1079/bjn19970104.

Borsheim, Elisabet, and Roald Bahr. "Effect of Exercise Intensity, Duration and Mode on Post-Exercise Oxygen Consumption." *Sports Medicine* 33, no. 14 (2003): 1037–60. doi: 10.2165/00007256-200333140-00002.

Fung, Jason. "Fasting and Muscle Mass—Fasting Part 15." *Intensive Dietary Management*, October 9, 2015. https://intensivedietarymanagement.com/fasting-and-muscle-mass-fasting-part-14/.

Garnier, P., F. Raynaud, and J. C. Job. "Growth Hormone Secretion during Sleep." *Hormone Research Horm Res* 29, no. 4 (1988): 133–39. doi: 10.1159/000180989.

Godfrey, Richard J., Zahra Madgwick, and Gregory P. Whyte. "The Exercise-Induced Growth Hormone Response in Athletes." *Sports Medicine* 33, no. 8 (2003): 599–613. doi: 10.2165/00007256-200333080-00005.

Halberg, N. "Effect of Intermittent Fasting and Refeeding on Insulin Action in Healthy Men." *Journal of Applied Physiology* 99, no. 6 (December 1, 2005): 2128–36. doi:10.1152/japplphysiol.00683.2005.

Henson, Lindsey C., and David Heber. "Whole Body Protein Breakdown Rates and Hormonal Adaptation in Fasted Obese Subjects." *The Journal of Clinical Endocrinology & Metabolism* 57, no. 2 (1983): 316–19. doi: 10.1210/jcem-57-2-316.

Klabunde, Richard E. "Hemodynamics of a Valsalva Maneuver." *Cardiovascular Physiology Concepts*, April 28, 2014. http://www.cvphysiology.com/Hemodynamics/H014.htm.

Klein, S., O. B. Holland, and R. R. Wolfe. "Importance of Blood Glucose Concentration in Regulating Lipolysis during Fasting in Humans." *The American Journal of Physiology* 32, no. 9 (January 1990): 258.

Liu, J. J., M. Crous-Bou, E. Giovannucci, and I. De Vivo. "Coffee Consumption Is Positively Associated with Longer Leukocyte Telomere Length in the Nurses Health Study." *Journal of Nutrition* 146, no. 7 (2016): 1373–78. doi: 10.3945/jn.116.230490.

"Macronutrients: The Importance of Carbohydrate, Protein, and Fat." McKinley Health Center, February 4, 2014. http://www.mckinley.illinois.edu/handouts/macronutrients.htm.

Martin, William, Lawrence Armstrong, and Nancy Rodriguez. "Dietary Protein Intake and Renal Function." *Clinical Nutrition: The Interface Between Metabolism, Diet, and Disease* (September 20, 2005): 121–40. doi: 10.1201/b16308-10.

"Micronutrient Facts." Centers for Disease Control and Prevention, March 31, 2015. http://www.cdc.gov/immpact/micronutrients/.

Norrelund, H., K. S. Nair, J. O. L. Jorgensen, J. S. Christiansen, and N. Moller. "The Protein-Retaining Effects of Growth Hormone during Fasting Involve Inhibition of Muscle-Protein Breakdown." *Diabetes* 50, no. 1 (2001): 96–104. doi: 10.2337/diabetes.50.1.96.

O'Connor, Anahad. "Fasting Diets Are Gaining Acceptance." *Well*, March 7, 2016. http://well.blogs.nytimes.com/2016/03/07/ intermittent-fasting-diets-are-gaining-acceptance/?_r=3.

Proud, C. G. "Regulation of Protein Synthesis by Insulin." *Biochemical Society Transactions* 34, no. 2 (2006): 213. doi: 10.1042/ bst20060213.

Rothman, K. J. "BMI-Related Errors in the Measurement of Obesity." *International Journal of Obesity* 32 (2008). doi: 10.1038/ijo.2008.87.

Schoenfeld, Brad J., Zachary K. Pope, Franklin M. Benik, Garrett M. Hester, John Sellers, Josh L. Nooner, Jessica A. Schnaiter, Katherine E. Bond-Williams, Adrian S. Carter, Corbin L. Ross, Brandon L. Just, Menno Henselmans, and James W. Krieger. "Longer Interset Rest Periods Enhance Muscle Strength and Hypertrophy in Resistance-Trained Men." *Journal of Strength and Conditioning Research* 30, no. 7 (2016): 1805–12. doi: 10.1519/jsc.0000000000001272.

"Scientists Discover Hunger's Timekeeper." *Phys Org*, August 28, 2009. http://phys.org/news/2009-08-scientists-hunger-timekeeper. html.

Sisson, Mark. "Dear Mark: Women and Intermittent Fasting." *Marks Daily Apple*, June 19, 2012. http://www.marksdailyapple.com/ women-and-intermittent-fasting/#axzz2aeEOMKxC.

St-Onge, Marie-Pierre, and Dympna Gallagher. "Body Composition Changes with Aging: The Cause or the Result of Alterations in Metabolic Rate and Macronutrient Oxidation?" *Nutrition* 26, no. 2 (2010): 152–55. doi: 10.1016/j.nut.2009.07.004.

"What Is Your Body Type? Take Our Test!" Bodybuilding.com, 2014. http://www.bodybuilding.com/fun/becker3.htm.

ACKNOWLEDGMENTS

First and foremost, I would like to thank you, my reader, for your passion and interest in finally taking control of your life and finding freedom in fitness. To all the fans and readers of my blog HackYour.Fitness who have motivated and supported me: I look forward to continually serving you through the work I do.

I'd like to thank all the great influencers, thought leaders, and authors who I've had the pleasure of meeting and speaking with on this wild journey, each of whom inspired me to write this book in their own way: Derek Sivers, Gary Vaynerchuk, Tom Bilyeu, Dr. John Ratey, Ramit Sethi, Ryan Holiday, Pat Flynn, Chris Brogan, Hal Elrod, Nathan Chan, Chris Ducker, John Lee Dumas, and Lewis Howes.

Thank you to all the role models who were instrumental in shaping my fitness journey over the past 15 years: Arnold Schwarzenegger, Tony Robbins, Tim Ferriss, Tom Venuto, Tony Horton, Shaun T, Mark Rippetoe, Brad Pilon, Martin Berkhan, and Mike Matthews.

A big debt of gratitude to the entire team at Book in a Box including Tucker Max, Julie Stubblefield, Barbara Boyd, Caleb Kaiser, and in particular Zach Obront and Josh Raymer for their amazing patience and priceless advice. This book would never have been possible without their continuous support, guidance, backing, and help. Thanks to James Altucher and Marvin Liao for introducing me to Tucker and the brilliant business that helped me turn my idea into a book.

To my early Hacker team here in Hong Kong including Darryl O'Young, Wes Chu, and Timmy Chan: Thank you for being my guinea pigs.

Special thanks to Mark Jolley, my partner in crime. Sorry for boring you over all those cremas about this fitness stuff.

I'd also like to thank my family. Without their support, I can honestly say this book would never have seen the light of day. To my father who was a role model of courage and achievement from whom I learned the values of hard work and integrity. I miss you so much. To my mother who taught me the importance of love. To my brother Dan for calling me out on that hallowed day at the gym and kicking my ass into gear. This book all started from that little seed you planted in my head. To my amazing two daughters Laney and Jaime who were the catalysts in my life to begin this crazy journey and with whom I will spend more time with now that this book is finished!

Last but not least, this book is dedicated to my amazing wife and best friend, Ev, for her patience, her tireless meal prep, and her willingness to listen to my rants and raves about fitness, whether she actually liked it or not. Thank you for enduring all the early mornings, late evenings, weekends, and holidays that I was "working" just to make this book a reality. Thank you for pushing me and motivating me to achieve what I never thought was possible. I love you more than words can express.

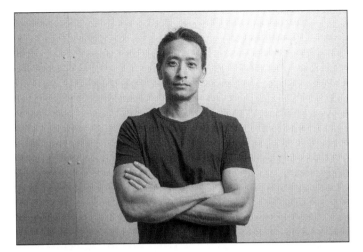

ABOUT THE AUTHOR

JAY KIM is a full-time investor and entrepreneur. He is the host of the popular podcast *The Jay Kim Show*, and the founder of Hack Your Fitness (http://hackyour.fitness), the complete fitness & lifestyle solution for busy professionals and entrepreneurs. He works with world-class athletes and other high performers to help them achieve fitness results that are sustainable for life. Jay is an active early-stage investor and avid supporter of the start-up ecosystem in Asia. Jay frequently consults with leaders in local government on topics related to technology, entrepreneurship, early-stage investing and startups. Originally from the Bay Area, he holds a Bachelor of Science in Business Administration from the University of North Carolina at Chapel Hill with a minor in Technology. Jay currently resides in Hong Kong with his wife Evelyn and two daughters Elena and Jaime. Reach out to him directly on Twitter @jaykimmer.

INDEX

B

C

D

traps 279
triceps 202, 208, 262, 276, 282
upper body 163, 201-4, *207,* 208-9, 262

F

fad diets 118-22, 126-27, 140
fasting, intermittent (IF) 89-111
   key takeaways 110-11
   action steps 111
   benefits of 93, 99-102, 111, 258
   body fat and 93, 95, 97-98, 110, 111, 231, 257-58
   definition of 94
   drawbacks of 102-3, 111
   as "fasting and feeding" schedule 94-98, 110-11, 258
   hunger and 96, 100, 101, 107, 108, 111
   metabolism and 93, 110, 257
   misinformation about 90, 91-93, 98, 110, 111, 258
   as optional 109, 111, 258
   protocols for 91, 104-9, 111, 258
   workouts and 97-98, 111, 242
fat (macronutrient)
   in balance with protein and carbs 118-19, 124-27, 133-34, 134t, 140-41, 258-59, 293
   examples 116, 130, 134t, 266t
   function in body 115-16
   Hack Your Diet guide and 119, 127, 134, 266-67, 266t
   restaurant food and 239-40
fat, body
   alcohol and 145-46, 150-51, 260
   burning of 93, 95, 97-98, 110-11, 135-37, 135t, 231-32, 258
   and cheat meals 231-32, 243, 251, 264
   correlated to calories 84, 85-86, 87, 123-24, 257
   measuring 81-82, 138-39, 141-42, 259
   and weight loss 227-28, 251, 264
   see also single-digit body fat
FatSecret.com 130
fear, dealing with 196, 211
Ferriss, Tim 23, 30
festivities, strategies for *see* social events during maintenance
fitness
   diet vs. exercise and 31, 62, 67-70, 70-71, 256
   industry, dishonesty of 26-28, 34, 72, 92-93, 110, 177
   as lifestyle change 29-34, 41-43, 255, 265
   log (app) 287-98
   as mental challenge 31, 34, 55-56, 255
   vanity and 17-23, 39-40, 43, 69, 180-81, 188-89

H

Habit Stacking (Scott)   46

habits, establishment of   46–48, 49, 56–57, 99, 142, 259

Hack Your Diet guide   119, 127, 134, 266–67, 266t

Hack Your Fitness overview   *see* fitness hack components

Hack Your Fitness Twelve-Week Workout Log   288t

"Hacker Friendly" meals   122, 128, 142

hangovers, help for   243–44

Harris-Benedict equation (for TDEE)   80–81

high bar squatting   284

high-intensity interval training (HIIT)   159–60, 161–62, 176, 231

hips, exercises for   194, 199, 204, 222, 263

Hofmekler, Ori   105–6

holy grail of fitness, key to   159, 183, 235

honesty with self

    about body's limitations   244

    about diet   67, 72, 230, 234, 253, 265

    about triggers   57, 234, 256

hormones   97, 101, 102

Hubbard, Orville   244

hunger

    "eating scripts" and   77–79, 96, 110

    intermittent fasting and   96, 100, 101, 107, 108, 111

    macronutrient tracking and   120–21, 140, 141

    workout schedule and   173, 233

hydrostatic weighing method   138, 139

I

IF (intermittent fasting)   *see* fasting, intermittent (IF)

imagery   53–56, 57, 198, 256

incline presses   *see* presses, incline

inflammation, reduction of   101

injuries, avoiding

    with bench presses   274

    with deadlifts   212, *214–15*, 218, 221, 222, 263

    with dips   283

    with good form   197

    through muscle memory   181, 196, 200

insulin sensitivity   96–98, 102, 111, 146

intermittent fasting (IF)   *see* fasting, intermittent (IF)

intimidation, at gym   166–67

introduction   *see* fitness hack (introduction)

IronMind   159, 178

isolation training   157–58, 166–67, 183, 201, 202, 248

Made in the USA
Columbia, SC
26 July 2020

14628085R00185